Health Secrets from the Orient

Other Books by the Author:

- *CARLSON WADE'S GOURMET HEALTH FOODS COOKBOOK*

- *HEALTH TONICS, ELIXIRS AND POTIONS FOR THE LOOK AND FEEL OF YOUTH*

- *HELPING YOUR HEALTH WITH ENZYMES*

- *MAGIC MINERALS: KEY TO BETTER HEALTH*

- *NATURAL AND FOLK REMEDIES*

- *NATURAL HORMONES: THE SECRET OF YOUTH-FUL HEALTH*

- *THE NATURAL LAWS OF HEALTHFUL LIVING: THE BIO-NATURE HEALTH RHYTHM PROGRAM*

Health Secrets
from the Orient

Carlson Wade

Foreword by WILLIAM S. KEEZER, M.D.

PARKER PUBLISHING COMPANY, INC.
WEST NYACK, NEW YORK

©1973, *by*
Parker Publishing Company, Inc.
West Nyack, New York

Library of Congress Cataloging in Publication Data

Wade, Carlson,
    Health secrets from the Orient.

    1. Folk medicine--East (Far East)   I.   Title.
RI33.W23   613   73-4917
ISBN 0-13-384552-4

PRINTED IN THE UNITED STATES OF AMERICA

Foreword
by a Doctor of Medicine

Here is the book for the layman as well as for the physician who is seeking to discover the secrets of Oriental health and longevity. This book is a treasury of hundreds upon hundreds of these secrets, taken from "forbidden scrolls," from the inaccessible regions of Tibet, from the herbal pharmacies of China, from the many nations of the past and present throughout the Middle, Near and Far East. At long last, Carlson Wade has probed many centuries of Oriental secrets and compiled them in this fascinating, helpful and beneficial book.

He has gathered these all-natural secrets from the Orient and presented them to the reader in simple, easy to use form. This enables the reader to follow the Oriental remedies right in his own home. The programs are all-natural, since the Orientals looked to Nature-created substances for healing. Carlson Wade shows how to use Oriental fasting, how to use healing plants available at your corner food market, how to follow "forever young" health secrets from the long-living people of Central Asia, how to use water, herbs, self-massage, fresh fruits and vegetables, seed oils, breathing exercises and honey, to help create the look and feel of youth.

Each chapter will offer a treasure of health rejuvenation secrets from the Orient. You are told how to rebuild youth "from the inside" with simple all-natural programs. You are shown how to restore the look of youth to your body with simple, yet reportedly beneficial Oriental secret remedies that take a few moments of time...and offer a "forever young" appearance of your skin, hair, eyes, arms and legs. The book is an Oriental treasure of health secrets taken from hundreds

5

of secret documents and reports, presented here in simple and easy-to-follow programs.

Carlson Wade does more than give you the Oriental secrets for youthful vitality and health. He tells you *how* these secrets can rebuild your body and mind. He tells you *why* these secrets can help you enjoy energetic-vitalic youth, as they have helped the privileged class of Orientals in the past centuries and right into modern times.

Carlson Wade has prepared a carefully researched and highly recommended book with personal impact and meaning for every reader who wants to experience the joys of youthful health...and who doesn't? The book is well-documented and an excellent home guide to better health the secret Oriental way. This book offers much help to those who seek natural healing, or who seek improved health using all-natural methods.

If you have ever wondered about getting the health secrets from the "forever healthy and forever young" Orientals, then this book will answer your questions. It will show you how you, too, can live better, live longer, live youthfully with these health secrets from the Oriental healers.

I highly recommend this book to those who want to know the successful Oriental way to prolonged youth and dynamic health.

William S. Keezer, M.D.

What This Book Can Do for You

For some 5,000 years, physicians throughout the Orient have reportedly been able to promote rejuvenation of the body and mind through the use of secret food combinations, herbs, special foods, massages, breathing exercises, simple water therapies and other health secrets. Ancient Oriental sages recorded these secrets in scrolls, parchments and documents that were kept sealed and hidden from the general populace; but as these miracle healings increased, the Oriental physicians slowly shared their secrets of "eternal youth" with other scholars who, in turn, revealed their own, once-jealously guarded healing secrets.

As the centuries rolled on, many of these health secrets were gathered together in Oriental scrolls and kept in private archives. Soon, the knowledge was shared by more "folk physicians," until the Orient became recognized as the place of "magic healing" through all-natural ingredients and methods.

I have devoted more than 15 years to the accumulation and study of secret writings and treasured natural remedies from all parts of the Orient. My research encompasses long-forgotten, out-of-print Oriental writings that cover a period of approximately 50 centuries. I have communicated and become friends with medical scholars from China, Japan, India, Tibet, Mongolia, Manchuria, the Philippines, Hawaii, Iran, Iraq, Thailand, Australia, Ceylon, and the many principalities throughout the South Pacific. These scholars, health practitioners and physicians kindly shared many of their acquired secrets with me. With this cache of natural healing secrets from the Orient, I embarked on an attempt to "bridge the gap" between East and West by contacting modern scientific laboratories, pharmacologists, physicians and chemotherapists. Their generously shared knowledge was further enhanced by my researching endless volumes of modern scientific journals, newly released interpretations of Oriental healing secrets and current medical treatises.

This treasure of Oriental remedies has now been painstakingly recorded and structured into this book. You have at your fingertips the result of all this research: a treasure of ancient healing secrets from the Orient that can be followed easily and applied in our modern times.

This book will show you how to help enjoy "eternal youth" by following the secret Oriental way of natural healing. The basic secret here is that the Oriental *treats the cause first and the symptom second*, to promote youthful healing. This book shows you how the hidden causes of many of today's common ailments can be alleviated and even healed by using natural Oriental health programs right in your own home.

Some of these do-it-yourself, easy-to-follow Oriental secrets will help you enjoy youthful vitality and extend the prime of your life; but this is only a starter. As you discover more and more secrets, you can share the Oriental way to:

- Rejuvenate your digestive system.
- Tap a hidden source of youthful energy.
- Help regulate your own blood pressure as a foundation of better health.
- Add years to your life by following the secret 10-step method of the centuries-young Central Asians.
- Relieve backaches and arthritic-like pains with do-it-yourself, Japanese *Shiatsu* treatments.
- Enjoy the virility of renewed youthfulness with "magic" substances that promote an extended sex life.
- Rejuvenate your mind healthfully and naturally with the Hindu *Prana* secrets revealed in this book.

These secrets, and many more, will be of benefit to those who are seeking the way to regain their youthfulness. They are presented in simple, do-it-yourself programs, without any special devices. Nearly all of the foods mentioned in these programs can be obtained at any nearby supermarket or health food store.

Within these pages you now possess the Oriental secrets of "eternal youthfulness" and lasting good health, as promised by the Asiatic and Eurasian physicians throughout 50 centuries of natural healing.

Carlson Wade

Table of Contents

Foreword by a Doctor of Medicine 6

What This Book Can Do for You 8

1. How Americans Can Benefit from Hidden
   Health Secrets of the Orient 17

The Secret of Oriental Folk Healers • The Secret Yin-Yang Method of Perpetual Youth and Health • The 12 Oriental Secrets for Health-Building • Secrets of Macrobiotic Diet Healing • How Ralph A. Used Macrobiotics to Help Alleviate Hypertension • How Arlene B. Used a Modified Macrobiotic Plan to Slim Down and Appear More Youthful • The Oriental Way of Health • Highlights of Chapter 1.

2. How Orientals Use Fasting to Promote
   Youthful Health and Longer Life 32

Oriental and Middle Eastern Fasting Secrets • How to Use a "Mediterranean Fast" in Your Own Home • Oriental Advice on Fasting Effectively • Secret of the Herbal Tea Fast • How a Modernized Liver Rejuvenation Fasting Program Can Work for You • In Review.

3. Oriental Secrets of Youthful Vitality
   from the Oceans 44

How an All-Natural Oriental "Fountain-of-Youth Cocktail" Promoted Overnight Rejuvenation for a Middle-Aged Woman • Orien-

tal Youth-Building Treasures Harvested from the Oceans • Secret Youth-Building Power of Sea Foods • How a Polynesian Tonic Gave Peter C. a Quick Rejuvenation Response • Ocean Plants Help Heal Arthritis Stiffness • "For Life and Health, Look to the Oceans" • Highlights.

4. How the Orientals Use Plants for Digestive Healing and Rejuvenation **56**

Secret Oriental Book of Plant Healers • How Oriental Plant Remedies Work • How "Barley Brew" Soothed a Housewife's Lifelong Indigestion • How a Herb-Fruit-Barley Healer Helped Establish Youthful Regularity • The Secret Internal Cleansing Action of the Apple • How an Ancient Apple Medicine Helped Heal a Schoolteacher's Stomach Spasms • How a Lemon Helps Heal Throat Disorders • How to Use a Lemon to Heal Foot Disorders • A Japanese Plant Healer for Poor Digestion • How an Everyday Plant Helps Cleanse the Kidneys and Bladder • How Berries Act as an All-Natural Digestive Purification Tonic • The Tibetan Clove Cocktail Youth Secret • Highlights.

5. How a Controlled Oriental Rice Diet Helps Regulate Blood Pressure the Natural Way **70**

Basic Health Benefits of Rice • The Favored Health-Building Rice of the Orient • The Oriental Way to Healthy Rice Cooking • Ten Secret Oriental Rice Fasting Programs to Help Balance Blood Pressure • How an Overworked Office Worker Benefited from the Rice-With-Fruit Fasting Program • How an Engineer Meets the Demands of His Job • How a Salesman Achieved Muscular Relaxation • How a Librarian Became Relaxed, Refreshed and Younger-Looking • How an Accountant Uses a Rice-Milk Fast for Rejuvenation • How Mona Rid Herself of Nervous Headaches and Blurred Vision • How a Factory Foreman Controls Hypertensive Outbursts • Main Points.

6. The Forever-Young Health Secrets from the Long-Living Abkhasians **86**

The Modern Land of Perpetual Youth and Health • Ten Health Secrets of the Abkhasians • In Review.

7. **Shiatsu: Secret Japanese Finger-Pressure Acupuncture for Natural Relief of Aches, Pains and Soreness** **93**

Do-It-Yourself Acupuncture Without Needles • How Shiatsu Helps Relieve Headaches and Neck Pains • How Michael U. Relieves Leg Aches With Shiatsu • How Irma V. Enjoys Relief of Backache With Simple Shiatsu • How Robert O'C. Uses Simple Shiatsu at Home to Ease Symptoms of Wrist and Arm Stiffness • The Secret Healing Power of Shiatsu • Summary.

8. **Secret Oriental Water Healers for Naturally Rejuvenated Health** **104**

How Orientals Help Ease Arthritis With Ocean Bathing • How Margaret McK. Helped Soothe Arthritic Pain With Ocean Bathing at Home • Alfred DeN. Feels "Young All Over" With Twice-Weekly Seaweed Baths • Mediterranean Secret of Youthful Skin • Special Highlights.

9. **Korean Ginseng: Magic Herb for Sexual Power** **114**

Love Potion, Revitalizer, Rejuvenator • Hailed as an Aphrodisiac • American Report on Ginseng • Soviet Union Praises Ginseng Powers • Reported Case Histories • A Doctor Tells of the Magic Healing Power of Ginseng • Different Ginseng Varieties for Your Use • Secret Oriental Formulae for Health Rejuvenation with Ginseng • A Modern Understanding of the "Secret" Rejuvenation Power of Ginseng • Highlights.

10. **Oriental Secrets of Youthfully Healthy Skin and Hair** **129**

16 Oriental Secrets of Using Salt as a Natural Youth Aid • How a Polynesian Airline Hostess Offered the Oriental Secret of Youth • How Orientals Use a Simple Fruit for Natural Rejuvenation • Ten Secrets of Using the Lemon as a Youth Restorative • The Oriental Herbal Face-Lift That Smoothes Away Wrinkles • Oriental Skin Exercises • How Orientals Use Simple but Rejuvenating Water Treatments • Summary.

11. The Hawaiian Fruits That Help Awaken and Rejuvenate the Digestive System 139

How the Papaya is Used as a Natural Fruit Medicine • Four Health Benefits of the Papaya Fruit • U.S. Government Praises the Health Values of the Papaya • How Papaya Helped Rejuvenate an Executive • Banana — The Simple Fruit With Magic Rejuvenation Powers • The Apple — Secret Youth Fruit of the Hawaiians • The Pineapple — Miracle Fruit of Youthful Digestion • The Melon — Nature's Secret Digestive Aid • How to Ease the Urge for Tobacco or Alcohol • Highlights.

12. The Miracle Vegetable Protein from the Orient — A Key to Forever-Young Vitality 153

Soybeans — A Meatless Source of Complete Protein • The Ten Youth-Building Powers of Lecithin in Soybeans • How Soybeans Gave Rose B. The Look and Feel of Youth • How Cooked Soybeans Offer Protein-Plus Benefits • How to Prepare Soybeans • Why Orientals Value Soybean Protein Above Meat Protein • Main Points.

13. Oriental Secrets of Toning the Heart for Youth and Health 164

How Orientals Rejuvenate Their Hearts With Plant or Fish Oils • How the Right Kind of "Oriental Fat" Helped Give Paul L. a New Lease on His Heart • The "Right" Fats and the "Wrong" Fats • The Oriental Way to Artery-Washing • The Yoga Breathing Exercise That Sends Healing Oxygen to the Heart • Doctors Report on the Heart-Health Benefits of Shavasan • Two Secrets of the Heart-Healthy Yogi • Important Points.

14. The Magic Healing Power of Tibetan Herbs 174

Youthful Healing from a Divine Source • Early Oriental Writings About Tibetan Youth Herbs • The Health Secrets of a 256 Year-Young Man • The Secret Tibetan Herb That Renews Cells and Tissues • Herb Secrets from the Monasteries of Tibet • How to Purchase Herbs • Summary.

15. **Oriental Reflexology: The Natural Way to Help Heal Muscular Aches and Pains** **185**

How Reflexology Soothes Muscles, Relaxes the Body, Stimulates Circulation and Induces Sleep • The 8 Secret Reflexology Motions That Help Melt Aches and Pains • How Gerald V. Uses Six-Minute Reflexology to Relieve Headaches and Refresh Tired Eyes • How Peggy J. Relieves Stiff Wrists With a Reflexology Secret from India • The Eight-Step Way to "Forever-Young" Arms and Legs • Important Points to Remember.

16. **How to Stay Younger Longer With Prana — The Hindu Secret of "Youth Breath"** **197**

The Three-Step "Total Relaxation" Hindu Secret • The Hindu Secret of "Youth Breath" Prana — In Eight Steps • How Prana Helped Ease Ulcer Distress • Prana Helps Rejuvenate an Aging Stomach • Summary.

17. **Honey: Health-Giving Secret from the Orient** **207**

The Honey Potion That Promised Rejuvenation • Oriental Secret' of Healing With Honey • How Honey Helps Heal Arthritis • Honey — Oriental Medicine from the Bee Hive • Highlights.

18. **The Oriental Secrets for Staying Youthfully Slim — Without Dieting** **216**

Japanese Nine-Step "Quick-Slim" Program • The Vitamin That Helps Keep You Slim and Perpetually Young • The Simple Hawaiian "Slim Bath" That "Melts" Fat from the Body • Control Your Appetite With Seaweed • How Orientals Enjoy a Sweet Food That Helps Keep Them Slim • How to Use Herbs To Wash Out Excess Weight-Causing Body Water • Seven Oriental Secrets of Eating to Help Remain Slim and Trim • In Review.

19. **Ancient Herb Secrets from the Orient for Modern Living** **226**

How Orientals Use Herbs for Healing • Oriental Herbs That You Can Use in Modern Times • Herbal Healing Secrets from the PEN-TS' AO KANG-MU • In Review.

**20. A Treasury of Oriental Health Secrets
and Folk Medicine** **234**

Oriental Methods of Relieving Disorders of: Arthritis • Respiratory and Circulatory Ailments • Aching Limbs • Kidney Disorders • Stomach Problems • Irregularity • Skin Blemishes • Allergies.

Index **245**

1

How Americans Can Benefit from Hidden Health Secrets of the Orient

A new health discovery is being made in our modern times: it is a treasure of hidden health secrets from the Orient. The discovery may be new to the western world, but to the forever youthful Orientals, it is a way of life and health that has kept them in remarkably alert vigor even up to the 80's and 90's. For hundreds of centuries, such health secrets remained in the hands of a select few royal physicians and folk healers; but gradually, as word of the amazing healing powers of all-natural programs and methods began to seep through the barriers, travelers and researchers have reported seeing as well as receiving such health treatments and recovering from ailments that "modern medicine" could only relieve.

The Secret of Oriental Folk Healers

Nearly all methods of Oriental folk healers use one basic "secret" program: heal the cause *first* and the symptom *second*. The Orientals have created a system of healing that is aimed at correcting the *cause* of a wide variety of health disorders; they reason that once the "disturbance" is corrected, then the *symptoms* can gradually cease and good health of mind and body is restored. This is the foundation for their healing pro-

17

grams. They have adhered to this belief through hundreds of centuries and have used all-natural programs that include fasting, corrective eating, finger-pressure acupuncture as well as standard acupuncture, healing massage, herbal potions and tonics, special "rejuvenation" plants and foods, and simple yet remarkably healing breathing exercises.

For thousands of years, the Orientals have been using their all-natural healing methods. Their people have developed remarkable resistance and a form of immunity to the ailments that have ravaged the people of the Western world. The Orientals have adhered to the "Golden Rule Of Health," which states that the body must maintain a "healing harmony" of balances in order to enjoy perpetual youth and health. Should any distress occur, Oriental healers immediately seek to restore the balance, correct the disruption and use all-natural methods to help bring about harmonious healing. All elements of Oriental healing are aimed at restoring this "healing harmony." The Orientals have also maintained that since the body is a creation of a divine deity, it must be treated with God-created natural methods and plants and foods. Since such all-natural methods have succeeded for so many thousands of years, we may well believe that this ancient health program of the East should be applied by the so-called modern practitioners of the West.

Why Natural Folk Healers Were More Effective than Oriental Physicians

The rulers of the many dynasties that dominated the separate nations of the Orient were most anxious to solidify their power. Often, they would appoint influential politicians or young students to posts of Official Court Doctors. Thus, the appointment of a man to a medical post was often a reward for a particular political favor and did not represent ability or knowledge. Furthermore, when these appointees were required to take official state examinations, they had to answer questions concerning such topics as philosophy, history and literature. Included within the tests were relatively few questions relating to medicine, and whatever medical information was included was enshrouded in theory and poetry. Many appointees had to pay expensively in order to take such tests and gain social position, titles and an influential office. It was considered poor politics for an appointee to fail such examinations after he had paid so much, and it was feared that failures would discourage other money-bringing appointees. So the examinations were more philosophical and cultural than medical, and out of this political structure, many incompetent men were given degrees as physicians.

The official physicians hardly practiced; if they did, it was to prescribe a simple tonic for a person of high social position. Because of the lack of skilled medical care in high Oriental society, the royalists and imperialists were constantly failing ill.

The Contrasting Good Health of Common People

The common people were treated by the so-called "folk healers." These were physicians who could not afford to take the state examinations, due to a lack of money and/or political influence. They were, however, well-trained as physicians and dedicated to healing. They used their knowledge in treating the poorer classes of the Orient and, in traveling among the poorer classes, they listened to traditional folk secrets, combined their medical skill with all-natural methods and were able to promote youthful healing among their patients.

The Rise of Family Secrets

The folk healers were rewarded with family secrets that had been handed down from generation to generation. The folk healers would blend these secrets with their skilled training and create healing miracles so impressive as to arouse jealousy among the court-appointed royal physicians. Fearing that the success of folk healing would harm their own social prestige and power, the royal physicians forbade the use of such programs. Thus began the rise of "family secrets," which became enshrouded in strict secrecy as a defense against the powerful royal doctors. Young folk healers passed on these secrets to the students they trained. A number of scrolls and works were written and kept closely guarded, lest they fall into the hands of the influential court physicians who would wreak havoc upon the dissenters. From generation to generation, from secret scrolls and writings, from word of mouth, the tradition of Oriental healing had its beginnings. It succeeded — it flourished — and it formed the basis of the inviolable rule of youthful health: help heal the cause *first* and the symptom *second*. This became a traditional art of natural healing that has since emerged as an important science in our modern times.

The Secret "Yin-Yang" Method of Perpetual Youth and Health

In the years 2697 to 2595 B.C., Emperor Huang-ti Nei Ching conceived of a circulatory system and internal arrangement that he divided into two basic principles: *Yin* and *Yang*. The Emperor (also called the Yellow Emperor because earth was designated as his patron element) noted that the human body was a duplicate of heaven and earth, and that it performed in a rhythm that promoted perpetual youth and health. He recorded his findings in one of the oldest written works on Oriental healing, which he entitled *The Yellow Emperor's Classic of Internal Medicine*. In this scroll (which was kept secret for hundreds of centuries and used only by a select few), the Emperor observed that perpetual youth and health could be achieved by maintaining a proper balance between the two separate elements of yin and yang. He went so far as to list functions, foods and conditions which were either yin or yang in nature, or a slight combination of both. Maintain a *balance,* noted the Emperor, and the secret of youth and health could well be yours.

The Meaning of Yin and Yang

Ancient Oriental healers believed that there was a constant struggle in the human body comparable to the same struggle in Nature between opposing forces. The fluctuations of these two polar forces, yin and yang, were said to influence universal energy and regulate the body's youth and health. The Oriental healers followed the basic principles of folk medicine by treating the *cause* of an illness through correcting this imbalance. Once the yin and yang principles were properly balanced, the *cause* of the ailment was said to be corrected and the *symptoms* subsided.

Today, in our modern knowledge, we know that the Oriental folk healers were ahead of their time in making this discovery of perpetual youth and health. We may not call these forces yin or yang; we may call them acidity or alkalinity, for example. However, despite cultural differences, the Orientals' discovery of these forces must be recognized as a significant scientific contribution.

The Health Influence of Yin

Yin signifies acid secretions in the digestive system and an expansion of its functions; it is considered a passive, cool, dark and somewhat receptive element. Yin-dominated body parts include the liver, heart, spleen, lungs and kidneys. Orientalists feel that disorders of these emotions or body parts indicate a disturbance in the yin factor.

The Health Influence of Yang

Yang signifies alkaline secretions in the digestive system and a soothing element; it is considered more actively healing, warm, bright and more independent. Yang-dominated body parts include the intestinal and bowel tracts, gall bladder, stomach and bladder. Orientalists feel that disorders of these emotions or body parts indicate a disturbance in the yang factor.

How Foods Can Help Regulate The Health-Building Yin-Yang Balance

Orientalists maintain that good health is a reward for regulating the yin-yang balance through common-sense eating of special foods. The folk healers, who managed to learn ot these secrets, used them for correcting disorders among the people. They created this amazingly simple, amazingly modern guide for helping to regulate the balance with simple eating practices. Today, the Orientalists have blended the ancient with the modern as a means of creating a basic set of 12 steps to a healthful yin-yang balance through judicious eating.

The 12 Oriental Secrets for Health-Building

As you read these 12 steps, note that they draw from thousands of years of folk healing and are balanced with our modern knowledge of good health:

1. In a cold (yin) climate, eat more grains, vegetables, fish and desired meats. In a warm (yang) climate, eat more fruits and vegetables and less of fish or meats. This helps establish a healthy balance in your digestive system and promotes more favorable assimilation.

2. Your foods should be as natural as possible. The modern Oriental folk healers are aware of chemicalized and industrialized foods and urge their followers to avoid them in order to help maintain the delicate yin-yang balance. They suggest eliminating all canned or bottled foods. The belief is that since the body is a child of Nature, it should be treated lovingly with foods created by Nature. Any deviation is a disturbance of the yin-yang balance and resultant ill health.

3. Your fruits or vegetables should be organic, insofar as these are available. Avoid those foods that have been tainted with chemical fertilizers or harsh insecticides. While the ancient Orientalists were better able to partake of organically grown foods and, thus, were free of this problem, modern people need to exercise care in selection of healthful food.

4. If you are tempted to eat spicy foods, select those that are very mild — they will bring less disturbance to this delicate yin-yang balance.

5. Your foods should be familiar to your climate and your environment. The Oriental healers feel that the yin-yang precision balance is best maintained when foods are in harmony with the immediate surroundings. If you must eat something exotic or different, just consume a small portion until you are able to adjust your harmony to this strange food.

6. All fruits and vegetables should be in season. The Oriental health secret is that seasonal fruits and vegetables are in harmony with the digestive-assimilative system and thus, they promote better yin-yang precision balance.

7. Unnatural beverages should be eliminated since they cause discord with the yin-yang balance. The Oriental folk healers feel that unnatural beverages (which would include coffee, soft drinks, alcoholic beverages, commercial teas) create an antagonistic reaction to the yin-yang balance. This disruption often results in worse-than-average health.

8. For tea drinking, select all-natural herbs. The commercial teas are usually dyed or chemically treated and this creates a volatile reaction to the delicate internal balance. The Oriental healers have always emphasized the sipping of all-natural, herbal teas, which are said to be soothing to the yin-yang balance.

9. Meats and fish should be organic. Modern folk healers have reported that many of their patients suffered a variety of illnesses because of excessive consumption of chemically treated meats and fish. When placed on an organic or natural meat and fish program, the sensitive yin-yang balance was restored and healing began to take place.

10. For persons troubled with impaired digestion, a folk healer would suggest that there be *no* liquids taken with meals. The Oriental folk healers explained that to "drown" the yin or the yang secretions in lots of water would dilute their effectiveness, thus impairing the assimilation of essential nutrients. Many folk healers urged their patients to eat their meals without imbibing in water or other copious liquids as a means of enabling the yin-yang secretions to digest foods in a soothing and healthful manner.

11. The problem of indigestion, or stomachache as we call it today, is regarded as a symptom of upset yin-yang balance by the Oriental healer. To alleviate this, it is suggested that you sip tepid liquids — neither too hot nor too cold, since either extreme is antagonistic to the polarized elements — *after* your meal. This is said to help soothe your elements and promote internal harmony. A cup of herbal tea, a coffee substitute or slightly heated vegetable juice is very beneficial to the digestive system and the yin-yang polarized elements.

12. The serenity of the Oriental while eating is a picture of healthy digestion. The folk healers urged their patients to chew slowly, chew carefully and savor all that is eaten and swallowed. Careful chewing is soothing to the yin-yang digestive balance. It was the spiritual leader, Mahatma Gandhi, who once said, "You must chew your drinks and drink your foods to help create a harmonious yin-yang balance."

The preceding 12 health secrets are drawn from many fragments and scrolls of folk healing documents that have endured throughout the centuries — and they are surprisingly modern in their benefits. While the ancient Orientals may have lacked our modern scientific laboratories, they possessed wisdom and common sense and were well ahead of their time in realizing that youthful health may be a possibility with the restoration of internal balance.

Basic Yin Foods

These foods are said to possess healing benefits that are soothing to the body organs influenced by the yin principle. Folk healers would suggest increased intake of these foods, with decreased intake of others, to help give the body its needed "yin food." Such foods are:

organic chicken	cucumber	orange
organic beef	beans	fig
sole	potato	banana
trout	sweet potato	grapefruit
halibut	tomato	mango
barley	eggplant	papaya
whole wheat	goat's milk	pineapple
corn	margarine	lime
rye	butter	molasses
oats	cream cheese	honey
red cabbage	sweet cream	peanut oil
celery	sour cream	safflower oil
green peas	yogurt	sunflower oil
garlic	peach	white sesame oil
mushroom	hazel nut	menthol
bamboo shoots	cashew nut	thyme
artichoke	peanut	deep well water
spinach	pear	fruit juices
asparagus	melon	

Basic Yang Foods

These foods are said to possess healing benefits that are soothing to the body organs influenced by the yang principle. Folk healers would suggest increased intake of these foods, with decreased intake of others, to help give the body its needed "yang food." Such foods are:

organic eggs	carrot	dutch cheese
organic turkey	pumpkin	roquefort cheese
sardine	parsley	apple
herring	radish	strawberry
salmon	onion	chestnut
buckwheat	turnip	cherry
millet	kale	sesame oil
natural brown rice	endive	ginseng tea
dandelion root	lettuce	mu tea
watercress	goat cheese	chicory

Secrets of Macrobiotic Diet Healing

Macrobiotics is a recent discovery of natural healing that was heretofore kept secret for fear it would be misused by unskilled people. Originally, it was created by a Japanese doctor, Dr. Sagen Isiduka, at the turn of the century. Dr. Isiduka developed a modern biochemical interpretation of the ancient Oriental yin-yang principle. He formulated a set of secret rules for better living that were aimed at helping to restore this precision balance of healing.

"Macrobiotics" is concerned with wholeness and with perpetual youth and health; it offers a wholesome life of vigor and creativity. The secret is to help re-establish balance in an individual who has become either too yin or too yang. Dr. Isiduka explained that the body is influenced by the two forces of Nature:

> *Yin* — passive, centripetal, delicate.
> *Yang* — positive, centrifugal, aggressive.

Macrobiotics is aimed at helping to reset this balance, which may have become disrupted by errors in living. Dr. Isiduka created a program to help promote a natural healing process in a few of his chosen patients. He had hoped to keep his discovery a secret so that it could not be misinterpreted or erroneously used by others, but his healing successes were so great that word spread throughout the Orient until he reportedly was able to cure some hundreds of thousands of people by this all-natural method. Soon, macrobiotics was spoken of in the Orient as a miracle healing plan.

Dr. Isiduka was successful because he promoted health through nutritional principles and treated the *cause* as a means of healing the *symptom*. He finally revealed his secrets to another Japanese doctor, Dr. George Ohsawa, who became his successor. Dr. Ohsawa has continued to blend the ancient with the modern to come up with a workable method of promoting healing through macrobiotics. (The term "macrobiotics" was termed by Dr. George Ohsawa (Sakurazawa Nyoiti), who was raised as a Westernized Japanese, hence his skillful blending of folk healing with modern science. The word is derived from the Greek: *macro* means great, *bio* means vitality and *biotics,* that which gives vitality. Macrobiotics, according to Dr. Ohsawa, is the ancient modern technique of selecting and preparing food in order to promote a yin-yang balance that will lead to longevity and rejuvenation.)

Modern Scientific Interpretation

Dr. Ohsawa created a list of seven basic secrets for macrobiotic healing. These are based on emphasizing either the yin or the yang foods (listed previously) for healing of the influenced organs and conditions (also listed previously). Dr. Ohsawa treated several thousand patients by selecting healing foods for their yin or yang influence and by prescribing the following seven basic secrets of all-natural healing:

Secret #1. *Eat foods that are pure, whole and natural.* All foods should be as natural as possible, and as close to their natural state as possible. Avoid processed, canned and chemicalized foods. If possible, you could grind your own flours from unbleached grains. Soups should be made from natural vegetables and organic meats or fish. Avoid processed mixes or artificial flavorings.

Secret #2. *Select foods that grow and thrive naturally in your local area and eat them in season.* All foods should be of a natural source. If a food cannot be grown in your climatic region or is out of season, it should be eliminated because it may be responsible for upsetting your yin-yang balance.

Secret #3. *Chew all of your foods and sip all of your liquids.* Chew your foods to help stimulate the digestive processes and thereby promote better assimilation. Enzymes are sent forth to promote better digestion when foods are chewed and when liquids are sipped. Never gulp down your food. Proper chewing will help bring about a soothing yin-yang balance and promote a feeling of lightness and energy.

Secret #4. *Eating should be enjoyed in a climate of healthful hunger and not on a time-clock schedule.* Hunger is Nature's signal for food intake. (It is said to be a gift of the Oriental deities.) The Orientals note that without hunger, the blood is still concentrated in the lower regions, and it may cause a digestive burden to call forth more blood during eating. An essential secret of macrobiotic healing is to eat only when hungry, instead of adhering to a time-clock schedule.

Secret #5. *When you eat, reflect Oriental serenity and express silent gratitude for your food.* The delicate yin-yang balance becomes sharply upset during times of fatigue, anger or upset. The macrobiotic healer observes that eating under such adverse conditions will affect the quality of the food, disrupt the balance and create ill health. It is wise to be serene and grateful. A moment of meditation is emotionally soothing and promotes better assimilation.

Secret #6. *Eat two meals a day.* The amazing vitality of many Orientals may be in this health secret, which is one of the essential principles of macrobiotic healing. Eat just two meals a day: your breakfast should be enjoyed in the morning, after you have permitted your body time to awaken and become receptive to the foods it is to be given; your larger meal should be much later in the day — but at least five hours *before* bedtime. Macrobiotic folk healers say that the yin-yang balance is more precision-timed when you allow plenty of time for your stomach to be empty before sleeping. This is said to help induce a more deep and refreshing sleep.

Secret #7. *Be joyous in activity and exercise.* Keep yourself active. Macrobiotic followers were instructed to go to the beach, the mountains, the forests. They were told to breathe the pure clean air, to relish in the woods and streams. They were told to enjoy the feeling of gentle breezes and warming sunshine against the body. In particular, it was said that the yin-yang principle could be established when the body could enjoy the changes of the seasons without the need for excessive central heating or air-conditioning. "Enjoy the changes and flow with them. Experience the rising and setting of the sun and moon," was one of the doctor's suggestions for better internal harmony.

The art of macrobiotics calls for living as close to Nature as possible. Dr. Ohsawa reportedly has healed thousands of people of their infirmities by using a skillful blending of ancient and modern folk programs under a macrobiotic method. Soon, his secrets became known and many followers and practitioners revealed them to the world. Successes continue to increase.

How Ralph A. Used Macrobiotics To Help Alleviate Hypertension

As an overworked businessman, Ralph A. was a heavy chain smoker, a chronic pill taker, habituated to one prescribed narcotic after another. He had an alarmingly high blood pressure reading; his face was flushed. He had severe heart palpitations, and his chronic hypertension threatened to severely affect his heart. Fearing for his life, Ralph A. began trying one program after another. He found a macrobiotic folk healer during a business trip to Tokyo, Japan, and he agreed to follow the Oriental healer's advice.

The Simple yet Effective Healing Program: The preceding seven secrets had to become part of Ralph's daily living program. He had to emphasize more yin-listed vegetables and decrease some of the yang foods, which were responsible for the internal unrest.

Benefits: It took up to two weeks of such careful living before Ralph A. began to feel better. He gave up smoking, eased up on his narcotics and was soon looking and feeling much better. The benefits, as explained by the macrobiotic folk healer, were these:

Health is achieved by creating a balance of the yin-yang elements. In Ralph, the yin element was his orthosympathetic force, which helped to dilate (expand) all tissues and organs of his body. His yang element, the parasympathetic force, was overwhelming in that it controlled constriction. Therefore, by emphasizing more yin foods and cutting down on yang foods, he was able to achieve the desired balance and enable a dilation of constricted tissues and organs and a smooth internal flow.

Yes, Ralph A. was able to become naturally relieved of hypertension and related disorders by correcting this imbalance.

How Arlene B. Enjoyed a Trim-Slim Figure and Youthful Appearance on a Modified Macrobiotic Plan

At age 40, Arlene B. looked much older. She was corpulent — plain fat. Her skin was sallow, and she was always tired. She could not resist eating all sorts of sweets and snacks, and diets did not work because they could not ease her obsessive urge to eat. Once she finished with a diet, Arlene B. immediately reverted to her chronic eating with the result that she not only gained back the pounds she had lost, but gained extra weight. She was resigned to obesity until a devoted friend told her how she, herself, had discovered a simple macrobiotic program that gave her taste satisfaction, appetite pleasure and helped her slim down at the same time.

Arlene B. followed the preceding seven secrets for macrobiotic healing.

Benefit: The yin-yang balance has to be restored as a foundation for whatever healing is then to occur. This is the starting point. Arlene B. then followed her friend's program that had helped her slim down. The simple program:

1. Breakfast consisted of a bowl of whole-grain, natural brown rice, with a spoonful of honey for sweet taste.

Benefit: Macrobiotic practitioners feel that brown rice is considered to be the most perfectly balanced yin-yang food. (The food proportion for a normal feeling of youthful health is usually 5 of yin to 1 of yang.) Brown rice should be thoroughly chewed — this helps satisfy the eating instinct. It is regarded as a perfect balance of alkalinity and acidity; hence, it stabilizes the delicate yin-yang balance and eases the eating compulsion. Brown rice is said to contain a natural balance of 5 parts potassium (yin) to 1 part natural sodium (yang), which creates a good health balance.

2. Mid-day, Arlene B. would enjoy a cup of natural herbal tea with a tablespoon of organic honey. The tea offered many nutrients as well as an expansive feeling, which eased the appetite, and the honey served to satisfy the sweet taste buds.

3. The main meal consisted of a combination of whole grain cereals (yang) with raw vegetables (yin) as a means of further balancing the healthful ratio.

4. As a late evening "appetite easer," she would have a bowl of vegetable soup made from the green parts of such foods as carrots, radishes and squash. The benefit here is that these normally discarded greens are prime sources of essential minerals that help create a healthful digestive process.

5. Salt was prohibited. The reason for this was that the potassium from the vegetables was needed to help create a better yin, and sodium was an excessive yang — hence, the overweight. By omitting salt, the yang could be lowered and the yin raised to a soothing balance.

6. After two days of this simple macrobiotic reducing program, Arlene B. could take more vegetables, some organic fish, fowl and some fruits. After one week, she could take some very lean organic meats. Portions were limited. Throughout the entire program, Arlene B. began each meal with a bowl of steamed natural brown rice.

Secret Benefit: The process of digestion caused the rice granules to expand; the natural cellulose became inflated and, thus, put a curb on the appetite. This promoted a natural feeling of fullness, and Arlene B. ate modestly, although she felt satisfied.

Within three weeks, Arlene B. slimmed down. Her complexion was radiant and her figure was neat and trim. She no longer felt nervous, she was no longer the victim of insomnia and she felt healthy and youthful. She looked the picture of slim youth, thanks to the Oriental secret of macrobiotic health through restoration of the yin-yang principle. Simple, yes. Effective, definitely!

The Oriental Way of Health

In the words of Dr. Georges Ohsawa, "Oriental philosophy is simply a practical discipline of life that everyone can observe with the greatest pleasure wherever and whenever one wishes. It restores at the same time health and harmony of mind, soul and body, which are essential for joyful living."

To the Oriental, youthful health is the reward for balanced health. This is created by adjusting the two opposing forces that confront each other in all aspects of Nature and circulate in the body in the form of vitality flowing along precisely determined lines. The distribution of this youth energy is often disturbed. When this occurs, the modern Oriental folk healer is called upon to help bring about a balance, create internal harmony and youthful health.

Throughout the hundreds of centuries, scores of scrolls, books and records were kept, detailing thousands of all-natural healing methods. Now, such healing methods are becoming part of our modern sciences and are being recognized as having valuable properties of health restoration.

HIGHLIGHTS OF CHAPTER 1:

1. Oriental folk healers were able to promote well-being and youthful health in their patients by using natural methods to restore the Yin-Yang balance wheel of good health.

2. Follow 12 simple steps to help create internal yin-yang balance.

3. Modern macrobiotics combines with ancient folk programs to help create healing through all-natural means.

4. A Japanese doctor has created seven basic secrets for macrobiotic healing that can be easily used in modern daily living.

5. A simple macrobiotic program healed Ralph A.'s hypertension and made him look and feel youthfully healthy.

6. A modified marcobiotic plan enables Arlene B. to slim down while satisfying her appetite.

2

How Orientals Use Fasting
to Promote Youthful Health
and Longer Life

An ancient Oriental health secret that has always been considered most rejuvenating and healthful is that of *fasting*. Indeed, when we refer to health secrets, we mean healing therapies that have been successful throughout the Orient, but hardly known or recognized in the Western countries of the world. Fasting is one such Oriental health "secret," in that it has been known to promote youthful healing amongst rejuvenation seekers throughout the East.

Fasting is a Traditional Oriental
Method of Rejuvenation

At the very dawn of civilization, there evolved a secret worship or "health-religion" known as the *Ancient Mysteries*. The wise men traveled throughout Egypt, India, Greece, Persia, Thrace, Scandinavia and the Gothic and Celtic nations. They prescribed periodic fasting as a means of self-cleansing the system, casting out noxious wastes, and promoting a feeling of youthful health and longer life.

These beliefs were adopted by the druidical religion of the Celts, which required that a member of the sect undergo a period of fasting before he could advance in religious stature. It was said that five days of total abstinence from solid food, but drinking fresh fruit and vegetable juices, would help restore the internal harmony needed to create coveted good health. A fast of fifty days was also required in the Mithriac religion in Persia. Indeed, fasting was a requirement to all the sects and was similar to the secrets of health that were practiced in Egypt.

The Mysteries of Tyre, which were present in Judea some 2,000 years ago in a secret society known as the *Essenes,* also prescribed fasting as a means of promoting youthful health. longevity and clear thought.

In the first century A.D., there existed in Egypt an ascetic sect called Therapeutae, whose members followed the fasting health rules of the Essenes, taking much from the Kabala and from the Pythagorean and Orphic systems. These Therapeutae created miracle healings among the afflicted by promoting fasts ranging from one day to one month. The fasts consisted of one day of solid food abstinence to one week or even one month of abolition of solid foods. The healers prescribed natural raw juices to help nourish and cleanse the body and to enable the organism to promote self-healing and a feeling of rejuvenation.

Fasting has always been used as a healing method among islanders of the Pacific, even before their contact with Buddhism (which incorporates regular fasting as a religious devotion). In Eastern Asia and wherever Brahmanism and Buddhism have spread, fasting has been looked upon as a secret method of rejuvenation. Today, we have come to regard fasting as a significant program for improving the look and feel of youth. It is a secret of the Orient that has become a natural healer in our modern times.

The Rejuvenation Fasting Secret
of the Middle East

In a small and exclusive health resort on the Persian Gulf, the elite of Europe and the United States are found to be undergoing regular rejuvenation fasting programs. The programs are considered secret because few other health resorts have yet to seize upon them as methods of therapy. They are highly successful and have helped promote a feeling of well-being in many who partake of these all-natural programs.

In a reported situation, Susan J. entered this health resort complaining of a variety of so-called "aging" problems. Internal toxemia had caused Susan's sallow complexion and stringy hair. She walked with a stooped gait and felt stiff of finger and limb. Her digestive abilities were so weak that whatever she ate gave her a burning sensation and poor assimilation. Susan J. exhibited all the symptoms of premature aging, even though she was in her very early 40's, so she placed herself under the complete supervision of the Oriental fasting specialists. Here is the rejuvenation program she underwent — one that can be undertaken right in your own home.

Two Day Self-Cleansing Preparation Diet. The Oriental healers prepared Susan J. for the fasting by putting her on a self-cleansing preparation diet. For two days, she ate only raw fruits or raw vegetables. The benefit here is that ingredients in raw fruits create a self-cleansing or "scrubbing" reaction in the system and help slough off much accumulated waste and debris in the system.

One-Day Internal Healing Program. Once the internal organs are cleansed, they are receptive to nutrients in fresh foods, which help promote tissue replenishment and cellular therapeutic healing. Susan J. was put on this simple, yet highly effective liquid program:

MORNING TEA: A cup of organic herbal tea, flavored with natural honey.

10:00 A.M.: A glass of freshly squeezed fresh fruit juice. Oriental healers have long known that juices have a medicinal value and are able to send a shower of healthful nutrients to the aging tissues and cells.

NOON: A glass of any freshly made raw vegetable juice, which may be flavored with a bit of kelp or sea salt.

3:00 P.M.: A cup of vegetable broth, mildly flavored with sea salt.

7:00 P.M.: A glass of freshly prepared vegetable juice.

NIGHTCAP: Before retiring, a glass of skim milk that has been simmered and flavored with natural honey.

Effects of the Rejuvenating Fasting Program

In the spirited tradition of Oriental healing, the internal harmony of the yin-yang balance can be restored solely through natural methods. Susan J. underwent the preceding simple, yet effective program for five days. After five days, she noted that her skin was bright and clear, her eyes were bright, her hair became thicker and luxuriant, and her weight was stabilized. Also, the improvement in her digestion allowed her to eat, enjoy and assimilate solid foods, and her troublesome irregularity (constipation) was relieved. Her posture improved and her joints became more flexible. In effect, Susan J. not only looked younger, but *felt* much younger than her 40 years — thanks to the revitalizing secret of fasting.

How to Use a "Mediterranean Fast" in Your Own Home to Boost Vitality and Youthful Health

Ceremonial fasting has long been a tradition among the Middle Eastern nomads and desert travelers; it is a part of their religion. Their natural law states that periodic fasting helps clear the mind and body and, thus, enables the person to enjoy the divine right of vitality and youthful health. Because of the preponderance of fruits in this Mediterranean region, many have found that a special fast using this luscious food can be most beneficial and healing. A Mediterranean Fast is tradition to these Middle Easterners. It can be a secret way to vitality and youth if followed in your own home. Here's the simple program:

Berry Juice Fast. For three days, drink freshly prepared seasonal berry juices. Begin with one glass in the morning, another glass at 10:00 A.M., repeat at noon, then mid-afternoon, and also as a nightcap.

Benefit: The vitamins, minerals and enzymes in the berry juice will help wash out the insides and promote a scrubbing-away of the toxins and wastes that inhibit tissue regeneration. Once the berry juice fast has succeeded in sloughing away debris, the cellular network is then able to use the collagen and enzymes offered by the juice for self-regeneration.

Raw Vegetable Juice Fast. In many of the health spas along the Mediterranean, guests are put on a raw vegetable juice fast as a means of promoting self-cleansing as well as introducing valuable minerals to the system. This is said to help restore the yin-yang balance and promote internal harmony, the key to youthful health.

In one reported case, Fred R. went on a special all-liquid fast for ten days. It is reported that during the fast, he had his urine examined and was told that he was eliminating high amounts of DDT and other deadly pesticide residues, which had been responsible for his ill health. Fred R. was diagnosed as having internal toxemia, but the controlled, raw vegetable juice fast was able to wash the stored-up pesticide residue out of his body.

The Amazing Results Fred Received

After a brief period on this Mediterranean raw vegetable juice fast, Fred R. reportedly experienced a feeling of energy flowing throughout his body. His eyes became clear; energy surged through his body. He was able to go up and down winding trailways in local mountainous regions and run with the vigor of a young desert nomad. The fast gave him so much vitality that he said he felt as if a tremendous burden had been lifted from his shoulders, and that he could "keep going" almost all day and much of the night. There is little doubt that this traditional fasting helped Fred R. enjoy a "second youth."

Oriental Advice on Fasting Effectively

The Orientals approach fasting with wisdom and tranquility. Many Orientals undertake fasting programs in their homes by following this simple, common-sense regimen:

1. Prepare yourself for the fast, both mentally and physically. Keep your work down to a minimum. Fast in a soothing environment that is conducive to the spiritual significance of this ancient healing art.

2. On your first day, *sip* your desired juices; savor each swallow. Be joyful in the delicious nectars which are replacing solids and are going to promote internal self-cleansing and a feeling of youthful agility.

3. On your second and third days of liquid fasting, be sure to take calming and soothing baths. The bath-water temperature should be tepid, since very hot water may increase your metabolism and upset the delicate balance created by fasting. Cleanliness is essential throughout the fast because body pores must be kept open in order that wastes may be washed out of the system.

4. When you end your fast, follow these important health rules:

- Break your fast by eating a whole sweet fruit; you may substitute this with a bowl of fresh vegetable broth or puree, without chemical spices or salts. Use herbs for flavoring.

- Gradually, add raw vegetables to your diet. Orientals prefer cooked beans because they are mild and soothing.

- Chew your food very thoroughly. Eat slowly. Allow your body to make the proper adjustment so that better assimilation is achieved.

- Take up to three days before resuming your regular eating program. Orientals are astute in knowing how to treat their bodies properly. Once fasting has promoted healing, they show their gratitude by rewarding their bodies with wholesome and natural foods. This is the Oriental expression of gratitude to the Divine Elements, which help promote a feeling of rejuvenation through fasting.

Why Fasting is the Oriental Secret of Rejuvenation

Although the ancients lacked our modern laboratory skills, they were far ahead of our modern practitioners in recognizing that the body must be "purged" of its accumulated wastes in order to help restore the yin-yang balance of health. Fasting is the Oriental secret of promoting this delicate balance and fostering a feeling of youthful health. Today, we know that fasting promotes these rejuvenating features:

1. Fasting creates the metabolic rejuvenation of autolysis (self-loosening), in which there is a self-disintegration of the body's waste substances.

2. Fasting helps liberate choked-up metabolism, freeing it so that the body's cells and tissues are able to draw upon the vital elements introduced via the fruits and vegetables taken during abstention.

The Oriental Secret in a Modern Interpretation

Oriental folk healers have regarded ill health as a symptom of internal imbalance. Practitioners have observed that infectious wastes, toxins and metabolic refuse can seize hold of the body's tissues, thus inhibiting their activity. Such toxins further slow up the body's processes and the various organs can lose their youthful efficiency. Accordingly, modern folk healers feel that the key to rejuvenation is to rid the body of these encumbrances. Their methods have been so successful that they became the secret of perpetual youth to those who underwent regular fasting and self-cleansing.

The Orientals have observed that several days of fasting will enable the various body organs (skin, kidneys, lungs, liver, heart) to function with greater vigor and youthful health. It has also been reported that regular fasting can lead to the expulsion of metabolic sediment in the form of offensive breath, intestinal eliminations, profuse perspiration, catarrhal disposals and darker urine (regarded as a symptom of release and expulsions of toxins). The Orientals felt that these substances were responsible for the upset yin-yang balance and, when cast out, internal harmony could then be possible.

In ancient times, many royalists would undergo a brief three-day fast prior to an important state or political function. The fast helped to normalize and stabilize their physiological-emotional organs and, thus, enable them to think with better clarity. The amazing and oft-enviable energy of the aged potentates of the Orient could well be traced to their secret fasting programs.

In modern language, we realize that the Orientals understood that *the benefit of a fast was to free metabolic action — the key to youth.* Body cells and tissues require nourishment for rejuvenation. They can be nourished only when impediments and sludges are removed. The fast helps cleanse out the toxic wastes because the only source of nutriment for these tissues is the internal debris. The cells are forced to "devour" these wastes, which are then eliminated by the body. It works when food intake is limited as a means of "forcing" the cells to draw upon these accumulations as the only immediate source of sustenance. Today, periodic fasting is recognized as the Oriental secret of internal rejuvenation and external health.

How a Herbal Tea Fast Helped
Heal a Royalist's Allergies

Tsang Kung, a well-known folk healer, was summoned to the estate of a well-known royalist, His Excellency, Master Hsin, Chief Supervisor of the Imperial Vaults. When he arrived, the folk healer saw that His Excellency was lying in his bed, surrounded by trays of sweet goodies and assorted confections. The folk healer was told that His Excellency had been suffering from high fevers, inability to breathe properly, coughing spells and general malaise.

Tsang Kung was asked to perform any of his "magic" to help heal His Excellency's distress. The folk doctor immediately ordered that all confections be removed. This was quite an affront to the royal physicians who had maintained that a sweet would help drive out the "sour spirits" that were responsible for the illness. But Tsang Kung explained that it was necessary to cleanse the system of His Excellency as a means of establishing internal harmony. He said that with the use of ordinary herbs, in the form of a comfortably hot tea, the "sour spirits" could be cast out and a healing force introduced within the body.

Because the royalist had a lifelong history of what we know today as allergies, he consented to any treatment, if only it would help relieve his chronic cold symptoms and feverish weakness. Folk healer Tsang Kung prescribed this simple allergy-healing program, although he did not, of course, identify it by its modern name.

How a Herbal Tea Fast Promoted Allergic Healing

A variety of different herbs were used to make steaming cups of tea. For three days, His Excellency, Master Hsin, was put on a simple fasting program. He was told to sip herbal tea throughout the day. No other form of nourishment, including solids, was permitted. Along with this, he was instructed to rest in bed.

Benefits: Herbal tea is able to conquer allergic fevers by means of a sudorific action; namely, it induces a form of healing perspiration. According to the ancient Oriental scrolls, a proper balance must be re-established among the inner organs in order to promote regeneration and healing. Herbs serve to introduce healing ingredients that help cast out toxins and metabolic wastes, which cause the internal imbalance. The fasting enabled the weakened organs to rest and regenerate, thus bolstering resistance to noxious allergy-causing substances.

Three Days of Fasting Promotes Lifelong Healing of Allergies

After three days of this simple, yet highly beneficial herbal fasting program, the noted Master Hsin was relieved of his fever, felt free and easy breathing, hardly coughed at all, and was eager to leave his bed and attend to his royal duties. He rewarded Dr. Tsang Kung, who returned to his people to help bring healing through Nature to those who could not afford a physician. It is recorded that these three days of herbal fasting promoted a lifelong freedom of allergies for His Excellency.

Secret of the Herbal Tea Fast

Dr. Tsang Kung was thousands of years ahead of his time. He knew that sweat-inducing herbs and controlled fasting would help expel the toxic wastes (evil spirits) from the body and thereby establish internal harmony and eventual healing. For thousands of years, folk healers have said that rich foods are often a major contributor to allergic distress as well as feverish colds. By eliminating the rich foods, and introducing herbal teas, the body is able to slough off the residues and promote healing harmony. The folk doctors have preceded our modern scientists, who hold the same view: restore the body's harmony through a herbal tea fast and there should be recovery. For if the person consumes an excess of food in the midst of illness, there is less hope of recovery.

Modern Herbs Help in Healing

Modern herbs, available from almost any health food shoppe or local herbal pharmacy, can help in the healing of allergic symptoms, just as they did in the bygone days of the Orient. Even today, Oriental healers will prescribe a program of fasting when there are symptoms of allergy, cold or fever. The herbs are to be brewed in the form of a tea and served as the only form of nourishment during the healing process. It is an ancient folk remedy that is highly recommended by our modern scientific practitioners.

How a Modernized "Liver Rejuvenation" Fasting Program Can Work for You

Throughout the centuries, traditional folk doctors have recognized the value of helping to rejuvenate the *ts'ang* (the internal organs, especially the liver). The Oriental awareness and knowledge of the structure of the human body was spread over vast areas of Asia, as well as the many islands of Japan. This awareness endured as irrefutable belief throughout the centuries, right up to our modern time.

Oriental knowledge of anatomy was the basis for the sixteenth century "discoveries" made by the European, Andreas Versalius, and his teachings about the workings of the human body. In particular, the Orientals developed a special "liver rejuvenation" fasting program. Many Oriental physicians wrote that such a program helped boost the health and the youthful vitality of their patients. It was said to help establish the precious yin-yang balance and thereby restore healing harmony.

This knowledge was applied by European scientists and has since been used in modern treatments with the same remarkable success. It is an all-natural program that is reportedly as effective in our modern times as in the days of the ancient folk physicians.

Here is how the modernized "liver rejuvenation" fasting program can help you:

PREPARE: A cup of fresh raw beet juice (use beets and greens. A special *Oriental Liver Tonic*. Combine 2 cups of fresh lemon juice with 2 quarts of water and 2 tablespoons of natural honey. Stir vigorously together.

FIRST DAY: 2 tablespoons of beet juice. One glass of the Oriental Liver Tonic.

SECOND DAY: 4 tablespoons of beet juice. One glass of the
Oriental Liver Tonic.

THIRD DAY: 6 tablespoons of beet juice. Three glasses of the
Oriental Liver Tonic.

FOURTH DAY: Drink freely of the beet juice and the Oriental
Liver Tonic throughout the day.

FIFTH DAY: Begin to break the fasting program by taking any
raw vegetable, grated, or raw juice in any amound desired. A
fresh raw fruit before bedtime is said to soothe the liver.

SIXTH DAY: Eat all you wish of raw ground seeds or nuts, and
all the raw vegetables or juices you desire.

SEVENTH DAY: Eat lightly of coddled eggs, sprouts, nut milk,
undercooked vegetables. A small portion of cottage cheese to
help begin your protein intake.

AFTERWARDS: Slowly begin a healthful eating program that
calls for low-fat foods with daily emphasis upon fresh raw fruits
and vegetables.

Suggestion: Oriental healers often prescribed *raw cucumbers*
as a means of establishing internal harmony and liver regeneration. Modern scientists approve because we know that raw
cucumbers contain an enzyme that helps to digest protein and
thereby provide better assimilation and healing of the liver and
other internal organs. Raw cucumbers may well be the secret
Oriental liver regeneration food.

Benefits of the Oriental Liver Rejuvenation Fasting Program:
The beet juice and special Oriental Liver Tonic help create the
aforementioned autolysis of the liver. This causes the process
of digestion or "self-loosing" of noxious wastes that have accumulated on the liver cells. Once these wastes are loosened and
cast off, the enzymes in the Oriental Liver Tonic are able to
nourish and regenerate the living and cleansed tissues of the
liver as well as other organs.

Thus, the Orientals realized that before the liver could be
regenerated it had to be "cleansed," and they prescribed the
aforementioned liver rejuvenation fasting program. What they
may have lacked in laboratory instruments, they did possess in
wisdom. They prescribed natural healing programs and recorded
the high rate of success among their patients, and they left a
rich legacy of anatomical charts and writings that showed how

astute they were in their knowledge of using Nature for healing processes.

If we compare our modern knowledge with the findings of the Oriental physicians over the past thousands of years, we can see that they approximate what we know to be actual fact. The folk healers of the Far East have spread their influence throughout the world. Today, we look to the East for knowledge and secrets of healing for our modern ailments and the quest for youthful health. One such secret is *fasting* — an ancient healing art that is becoming a modern "discovery" in the West.

IN REVIEW:

1. Youthful health and longer life were often rewarded to the ancients who underwent periodic fasting programs.
2. A simple rejuvenation fasting program, as used by guests at a health resort on the Persian Gulf, gave Susan J. a look and feel of perpetual youth. The very same program can be followed in the home.
3. A basic Oriental fasting program will help boost your emotional health. Follow the four-step program at your convenience.
4. A herbal tea fast (easily followed by anyone in our modern times) helped heal His Excellency, Master Hsin, of a lifetime of allergic distress. It took only three days.
5. *A Mediterranean Fast* in your own home cleanses your insides and promotes the yin-yang balance — the key to perpetual youth.
6. Fred R. enjoyed a raw vegetable juice fast, after which he looked and felt sparkling clean and alert. His previous ailments had subsided. He began to enjoy his "second youth" after the fast.
7. A modernized "liver rejuvenation" fasting program creates soothing harmony. Enjoy Oriental serenity and ageless youth with this time-tested folk program. It's all natural!

3

Oriental Secrets
of Youthful Vitality
from the Oceans

For thousands of years, the people of the Far East have harvested vegetables and sea foods from the rich gardens of the ocean. They have tapped many hidden secrets from the depths of the sea, and the rewards have been youthful vitality and energy. The Orientals have been able to build resistance to many of modern civilization's ailments by using the natural rejuvenation elements that flourish in the oceans and seas around them.

In an effort to discover the Oriental secrets of youthful vitality, our modern scientists have searched and researched the oceans and made discoveries that have been folk medicine for centuries to these youthfully healthy natives. Today, we are beginning to reap an ocean harvest of Oriental health secrets.

How an All-Natural Oriental "Fountain-of-Youth Cocktail"
Promoted Overnight Rejuvenation For A Middle-Aged Woman

Julia K. was under 50, yet looked older than the nurse-companion who had brought her to the Hawaiian seaside resort hotel. It was an extremely warm August day, yet Julia sat on a chair, cloaked in a heavy woolen robe, her knees covered with a blanket, while every door and window was tightly shut.

44

weight Orientals, and goiter is almost unknown. Senility is rare, arthritic limbs are rarely evident. Energy is manifest among the elderly, who are alert and active well up in their years, in contrast to Americans who are often "old" in their middle-age. The secret of such perpetual youth may well be in the treasures harvested from the oceans and used by the Orientals as part of their daily fare. Following are some of the harvested treasures from the oceans, which reportedly help promote youthful vitality among the Orientals.

Sea Plants

In the *Chinese Book of Poetry,* written almost 3000 years ago, there is a poem that describes a woman who cooks sea plants. Always considered a delicacy, sea plants were also offered up during sacrifices to the ancestors. Today, we know the plants as seaweed, a splendid source of minerals that help regulate the hormones, enrich the bloodstream, assist in metabolism, promote a youthful skin color, feed the shafts and ducts of the scalp to help improve the health of the hair, and help warm the body and promote mental youthfulness.

Seaweed has always been part of the staple diet of the Orientals, who lived near the sea and depended upon it for sustenance. It may well be the "secret" for a long and healthy life for you.

How To Use: Many health food shoppes and Oriental grocery houses sell seaweed in various forms. In dried form, it may be used as part of a raw vegetable salad or crumbled and sprinkled over a salad as a natural tangy seasoning. You might also use seaweed as a snack, together with a fresh, raw vegetable juice. You'll enjoy the full flavor of the sparkling oceans as well as the benefits of ocean-harvested vitamins and minerals.

In the Orient, seaweed is looked upon as a sexual stimulant and source of youth. It may well be the "secret" that the Western world has been seeking, but it has been known in the Orient for centuries.

Kelp Powder

A dehydrating process can reduce seaweed to a powder, which is a prime source of valuable thyroid gland-feeding iodine. Also, it contains a special beneficial *carbohydrate that does not raise the blood sugar;* instead, this kelp carbohydrate helps metabolize the protein, unsaturated fats and the many vitamins and minerals found in this powder so that there is beneficial assimilation.

Special Benefit: One type of seaweed, *agar agar,* available almost at all health food stores, helps to form a smooth, slippery bulk in the intestinal tract and acts as a natural regulator of the bowels. The absence of harsh laxatives in the Oriental way of life may well be due to their use of agar agar as a healthful and natural regulator. Many Orientals will boil agar agar into a jelly and use it as a base for soups or special puddings. It's considered a natural way to internal cleanliness; it may well be the best natural way to regularity and freedom from laxatives.

How to Use Kelp: Kelp powder is a healthful salt substitute. Use it in place of salt in almost all recipes. You might add some to your home baked breads, rolls, muffins, to help bolster their vitamin-mineral content.

How to Make a Stimulating Oriental Vigor Tonic

Mix one-half teaspoon of kelp in a glass of fresh vegetable juice. Add one-half teaspoon of agar agar. Stir vigorously. Drink early in the morning. The benefit here is that the minerals in the kelp combine with the vitamins and enzymes in the raw juice, then join with the natural nutrients in the agar agar to create a "morning energizer." The amazing and enviable vitality of the Orientals may well be due to the power of this all-natural Oriental Vigor Tonic. It's a popular morning beverage among modern Orientals and is regularly prescribed by their traditional folk doctors.

Algae

Algae are seaweed-like ocean plants with amazing health and youth-building benefits. Algae plants feed the glands and influence metabolism. Orientals who eat algae plants regularly are known for having very youthful skin textures. The reason is that nutrients in the algae influence the endocrine glands to *promote a healthful perspiration action.* This opens the skin pores, encourages sweating and casts out waste products (many of a fatty, unhealthful nature), thus helping to promote internal cleansing.

Special Benefit: When the internal viscera have been washed of debris, the algae are *then* able to deposit valuable ocean-born minerals onto the organs, rejuvenating and replenishing their cells and tissues. It is this exchange that is part of the *yin-yang balance of internal harmony:* cleanse out the debris, replace with sparkling fresh nutrients that regenerate vital youth-building organs! All this and much, much more from the ocean's secret youth food — *algae.*

How To Use Algae: Use algae as you would any vegetable substance. If you obtain it as a powder, use it as a salt substitute in baking, as well as for flavoring of foods. If you obtain it as a sea plant, use it as a vegetable in your raw salads, added to soups, or for tasteful and healthful snacks.

A Pacific Punch to Knock-Out
That Dragged-Out Feeling

In a glass of freshly prepared raw vegetable juices, sprinkle powdered algae. Stir vigorously; drink as a mid-afternoon "pick-me-up." The rich treasure of vitamins, minerals and enzymes works promptly to perk up a sluggish glandular system and give you a "punch" of vitality. It is said to be a daily beverage enjoyed by the hardy, youthful and energetic people of Hong Kong, and it can be enjoyed right in your own home.

Amazing Benefits of Ocean Fish Oils

Oils made from such fish as haddock, cod, shark, tuna, sardine, salmon and halibut are recognized as having superior health benefits. The Orientals are known for consuming a lot of fish and, when they also consume the oils, they are rewarded with clear skin, thick hair, a youthful circulation and a rich, red bloodstream.

Our modern scientists have discovered that the secret of Oriental freedom from arteriosclerotic-cholesterol problems may well be in fish oils. These liquids are prime sources of unsaturated fatty acids. An average serving is said to help neutralize the effects of saturated (hard) fatty acids and, thus, help reduce the blood cholesterol level. Since Orientals usually eat the whole fish, they also take in the polyunsaturated fish oils and thereby reduce the possibility of effects from excess cholesterol.

Modern research indicates that fish oils possess even greater amounts of polyunsaturated oil than do vegetable oils. The polyunsaturated portion of most fish oils is also more potent than that of seed or vegetable oils.

Secret Benefit: Seed or vegetable oils contain two or three "bonds" or linkages in the fatty acid, which are sites of unsaturation. The more bonds, the greater the unsaturated fatty acids. Fish oils contain up to six such bonds or linkages in a given fatty acid. As such, fish oils have an average polyunsaturation number of 5, in contrast to the low 2 or 3 level of unsaturation in seed or vegetable oils. The benefit here is that fish oils have a greater amount of polyunsaturated fatty acids, *which help melt cholesterol deposits* and maintain a free-flowing bloodstream. The regular consumption of fish and fish oils by Orientals may be the reason for their youthful agility even in their later years.

How To Use: Select fish oils from your corner market or health food store. Obtain a natural and organic fish oil for maximum benefit. Use in baking, as a butter substitute. Mix oil with some freshly squeezed lemon juice and a half spoon of honey for a truly delicious salad dressing. Use oil in almost any recipe calling for "fat."

Youth Oil Elixir: Pour two tablespoons of any fish oil into a glass of freshly prepared tomato juice. Add one-quarter teaspoon of kelp. Stir vigorously. Drink one glass about an hour after your main meal. The benefit here is that the vitamins, minerals, enzymes and the unsaturated fatty acids will help promote better digestion and assimilation of protein, and help disperse cholesterol during the metabolic process. In many fashionable Oriental hotels, a Youth Oil Elixir is considered a standard "after dinner" drink. It's natural — it's healthy — it's an ocean-borne source of perpetual vigor.

Fresh Fish

Because the oceans surrounding many Oriental nations are teeming with fish, it is obvious that seafood is part of their regular diet. Fish is the ocean's treasure of youth-building protein. Fish protein has many valuable amino acids, which are used to build and rebuild the body from inside to outside. Some 90 to 100 per cent of fish protein is digestible.

Special Benefit: Since fishery products contain low amounts of connective tissue and fibrous components, they are especially suited for low-bulk, bland diets. The amazing freedom from digestive disturbances for many Orientals may be in their habitual use of fresh fish, which is soothing as well as youthfully nutritious.

How to Prepare Fish for the Best Health Benefits

Obtain fish from health food shoppes or available organic food outlets. To prepare, take a tip from the Orientals: cook fish only until the flesh "sets" and can be easily flaked from the bones. The flesh of the fish may be likened to egg white and treated with the same delicacy. Fish may be baked, broiled boiled or steamed. The modern Orientals have this rule of thumb: fatty fish is broiled or baked; lean fish is broiled, boiled or steamed. The important Oriental rule to remember is *to avoid overcooking,* since overcooking can weaken the natural texture and flavor.

Special Tip: When cooking fish, use fish oils to further enhance their valuable health-building substances.

Secret Youth-Building Power of Sea Foods

The Orientals have long been aware of the secret youth-building power that is available through the consumption of fish, fish oils and ocean plants. While they may not have been able to scientifically identify the secret source of such health-building powers, they noted that fish foods made them robust, youthful and vigor. Our modern scientists have researched this secret and come up with this "magic" youth building discovery:

Magic Youth-Building Plankton

Infinitesimal ocean organisms known as plankton (from a mixed Greek-Oriental-Mediterranean word meaning "wanderer"), drift wherever the tides take them. These organisms form the food of many fish, however, the tiny plankton floaters are prime sources of ocean-nourished protein, vitamins, special carbohydrates and minerals, which are also valuable to humans.

Plankton is considered to be a "complete" food. Although plankton organisms have wandered throughout the oceans for centuries, it is only recently that science has recognized their magical youth-building powers. Also, it is now known that seafoods from the depths of the salt water oceans are prime sources of good health because of their intake of plankton — a magic youth-building ocean organism which can become the "complete" food.

Whether in the form of oil, whole fish or sea vegetables, seafood is considered to be a magic youth-building food by the Orientals. It is certainly one of the most important health secrets from the Orient.

How a Polynesian Youth Food
Helped Promote Quick Rejuvenation

The Polynesian peoples are known to enjoy a longer lifespan than the proverbial "three-score-and-ten years." These healthy, vigorous and youthfully alert South Pacific natives enjoy a long life that is comparatively free of the infirmities of Western civilization. While much of their "forever young" vitality is due to their clean, outdoor living, it is also known that they experience an upsurge of vitality by taking a simple "youth food." This youth food is known as kelp, the sea plant that is available in the form of crisp dehydrated leaves, or in the form of a special dehydrated white powder that contains the ocean's rich treasure of secret rejuvenating elements. To the Polynesian, a daily supply of kelp is the secret of his eternal vitality.

How a Polynesian Tonic Gave Peter C.
a Quick Rejuvenation Response

In a reported situation, Peter C., well up in his years, had been so ailing that he was bedfast. He had arthritis so severe that he could not even cross his legs. He became so disorganized that he could not remember his whereabouts at times! He could not feed himself. Many of his family members and friends gave him up for lost.

Simple Polynesian Tonic Promotes
Instant Rejuvenation

It was a simple, yet magically effective change in his regimen that brought Peter C. back from the lost. He was given a very simple Polynesian Tonic: one daily spoonful of organic kelp powder, dissolved in a glass of fresh vegetable juice. Within a few days, Peter C. got up from bed, was able to walk to the table, could cross his arthritic legs over one another and could remove his shoes. Peter's so-called "senile" symptons began to subside. Before long, he became so rejuvenated, he could hardly believe that he had ever been bedridden. Peter's mind and body were young . . . thanks to this traditional Polynesian Tonic.

The Magic Power of the Polynesian Tonic: A combination of enzymes and minerals in the tonic work to seize hold of the kelp's iodine supply. This supply is then soaked up like a sponge by the thyroid gland. Almost immediately, the thyroxin hormone is sent shooting throughout the bloodstream, regenerating the blood cells, helping to alert and awaken sluggish body metabolic processes. Once this happens, the body processes begin to rejuvenate. The ingredients in the tonic help to boost energy, overcome lethargy, send a warmth to the fingers and toes, stabilize a sluggish pulse, provide a balanced blood pressure and promote a general feeling of well-being.

So valuable is the need for "hormone food," such as that found in the Polynesian tonic, that a slight shortage could create internal havoc for a person. Ill health, with the debilitating, premature aging symptoms such as those noticed in Peter C., may be the consequence. Yet, the tonic's power — is so great that several days' use of the tonic is regarded as "youthful" by the forever-young Polynesians. It may be considered a modern discovery by the West, but it is a time-tested, centuries-old youth tonic from the wise folks of the East.

Ocean Plants Help Heal Arthritis Stiffness

In a reported situation, Helen E., a woman veterinarian, was subjected to wracking pains in the knuckles of her hands and also stiffness in her legs and ankles. She developed arthritic symptoms that so debilitated her, she had to give up her profession because she could hardly move her limbs.

Helen Tries Oriental Folk Programs

Hearing of the agility of the Orientals and learning of their traditional use of ocean foods, Helen E. decided to follow a home program based on the Oriental emphasis upon ocean plants and foods. Here is the program that Helen E. followed:

1. All oils were from a fish source. She would use fish oils for baking, for any recipe calling for oil and as part of a salad dressing. She used a variety of different fish oils, available at most health food shoppes as well as some supermarkets.

2. Daily, she would mix and drink a simple mid-afternoon tonic — one-half teaspoon of kelp in a glass of fresh vegetable juice.

3. She would eat fresh fish at least three times per week. She would bake, broil or boil the fish in some fish oil and season with kelp to further improve her vitamin-mineral-enzyme supply.

4. Nightly, she would make a raw vegetable salad comprised of algae and crisp seaweed. This would be flavored with lemon juice and fish oil, and a dab of apple cider vinegar for a tangy taste treat. Often, this raw seaweed salad would have fresh, raw vegetables as well. It was a delicious way to boost her health and emulate the ocean-worshiping faith of the Orientals.

5. She eliminated the intake of artificial foods such as cakes, coffee and soda drinks, and followed a more natural food program.

It is reported that this ocean-food program was followed for less than one year. Her arthritic stiffness melted away and she began to look and feel youthful. In a short time, she could resume her work, for her arms and legs began to move with characteristic Oriental ease and agility.

"For Life and Health, Look to the Oceans"

The ancient folk practitioners urged their followers to use the foods of the oceans to help lengthen life and rejuvenate health. Centuries ago, they recognized that the oceans abound with sources of healing seafood, whether in the form of seaweed or fish.

Today, we understand that the sea's resources do, indeed, yield a secret treasure of health. Many claim that ocean foods are more healing than land foods; this may be more than just an opinion. The rains and floods, prompted by wind, gravity and tidal waves, carry land's topsoil into the ocean. This top-soil is a prime source of vitamins, minerals, proteins, enzymes and many unidentified healing organisms. Yet, all go into the sea where they are naturally recycled in the form of ocean foods, waiting to be reclaimed. The sea may well be the world's source of life and health. The Orientals have always thrived because of the hidden secrets of health-building ocean foods. Now, those secrets are made available to you, to help you enjoy longer life and better health.

HIGHLIGHTS:

1. Oriental folk doctors have prescribed ocean plants and foods to help promote a feeling of perpetual rejuvenation.
2. The "Oriental Fountain-of-Youth Cocktail" helped promote overnight rejuvenation for Julia K.
3. The oceans offer a harvest of healing foods such as sea plants, kelp powder, agar agar, algae, fish oils and fresh fish — rich sources of health-building elements.
4. The amazing energy of aging Orientals may be due to the "magical ingredients" in the all-natural Oriental vigor tonic. It's regularly prescribed by traditional folk doctors throughout the Orient.
5. To help spark up sluggish glands, try a Hong Kong-created, all-natural Pacific punch as a mid-afternoon power-charger.
6. In many fashionable Oriental hotels, a youth-oil elixir is considered a staple "after dinner" drink. It's an ocean-borne source of perpetual vigor.
7. A homemade Polynesian Tonic helped Peter C. recover from months of arthritic-like pain and bedridden confinement.
8. A five-step program enabled "crippled" Helen E. to resume her normal activities. The program is based upon the Oriental "ocean-healing" seafood nourishment.

4

How the Orientals Use Plants
for Digestive Healing
and Rejuvenation

Some five thousand years ago, the Emperor Shen Nung taught his followers how to plant and harvest foods that were to be used for healing. He appears to have enjoyed a long and healthful life from the secret rejuvenation powers of special foods, because records indicate that Emperor Shen Nung lived to the healthy age of 140 years. During his lifetime, the Emperor traveled throughout most of Asia, visiting such areas as Japan, Mongolia, Manchuria, Thailand, Iran, Iraq and some of the Philippines, as well as certain regions of India. It is believed that he approached Tibet, and, while unable to enter, did meet with the sacred lamas, who ventured down from their sacred peaks to confer with his royal personage. Emperor Shen Nung devoted his lengthy life span to the gathering of these Asiatic secrets of using plants for digestive healing and basic rejuvenation.

Secret Oriental Book of Plant Healers

The Emperor compiled a listing of healing plants and described their rejuvenating benefits. The secret Oriental book, *Shen Nung Pen-ts' ao Ching (Pharmacopoeia of Shen Nung),* contained close to 400 different plant medicaments, together with some guiding principles for their judicious use. Because the all-natural plant remedies promoted such well-being and re-portedly healed many hitherto "incurable" ailments, the Em-peror kept his book a closely guarded treasure. He did not want adversaries to learn of his secrets. He applied the folklore reme-dies to himself and to a chosen few with the reported benefit that nearly all of them lived well beyond their hundredth year. Most important, they lived youthfully and with few of the so-called ailments of advanced age. Their use of plants for healing (the same plants that are available at almost every local super-market for a modest cost) helped rejuvenate their digestive sys-stems and promoted a variety of healing benefits. They were, indeed, rewarded with a long and youthfully healthy lifespan — thanks to the secret Oriental book.

More Asiatic Secrets of Rejuvenation Through Plant Healing

Knowledge of medicinal plants began to seep through the guarded vaults, in which many scrolls were kept hidden. Soon, other folk healers prepared collections of secret rejuvenation remedies. The great Pien Ch'ueh, some 2,000 years ago, wrote about a variety of plants that could be used to correct the dis-turbed yin-yang balance and restore digestive youth. In the 2nd Century A.D., a folk physician, Chang Chung-ching, created a scroll that listed plant medicaments to relieve problems of fe-ver, create a natural diuretic action, sedatives and body-toning plants, as well as emetics. Another folk doctor, Hua T'o, trav-eled throughout much of what is known today as Asia Minor and the Middle East, gathering traditional healing secrets that were handed down by word of mouth, from generation to gen-eration. He, too, compiled them in a set of parchment scrolls that were carefully preserved in hidden royal archives. Their secrets were given to favored royal personages and to visiting Asiatic rulers from whom favors were sought. Gradually, their secrets seeped out.

By the Seventh Century A.D. (the start of the Tang period, the peak of Buddhist influence), the first Asiatic medical school was created and a medical library of folk healers was established. One of the most prominent practitioners, Dr. Sun Szu-miao, had such success in using plants for digestive healing and rejuvenation, that the reigning emperors bestowed upon him the title of honor, "King of Plant Healers" *(Yao-wang)*. The folk physician compiled a precious collection of all-natural healing secrets in a work entitled, *A Thousand Ducat Prescriptions (Ch'ien Ching Fang)*. This work has been a valuable source of Asiatic secrets of rejuvenation and perpetual health through the use of plants such as fruits, vegetables and herbs.

Another immortal folk physician, Li Shih-chen, who lived during the latter years of the 16th Century, compiled a special *Pharmacopoeia (Pen-ts' ao Kang-mu)* in which he listed close to 2,000 different all-natural plant healers. The work included many of his own discoveries and compilations of hitherto forbidden and secret scrolls. Others followed in his footsteps throughout the centuries and, today, we know many of these previously guarded secrets. These discoveries were based on more than just traditional hearsay. Instead, these folk physicians used plant medicines throughout Asia and reported amazing success in helping ailing people to achieve healing and long life.

From these once-forbidden scrolls and works, we have a collection of reported successful treatments for the digestive system, as well as for the entire body. The Asiatic folk physicians devoted many centuries to the gathering of these priceless treasures and brought life and health to countless people. When we consider that the secret Shen Nung work, *Pents'ao Kang-mu (General Compendium of Remedies)* has nearly 12,000 prescriptions and formulas consisting of all-natural healing programs gathered from all over Asia and Asia Minor, we may truly agree with the Orientals that such programs are the "secret key to perpetual life and health." They worked for the tens of thousands who were healed; they may very well work for modern folks. Indeed, in the modern Orient, many of these secret remedies are helping to promote healing and well-being the natural way.

How Oriental Plant Remedies Work

The Oriental plant remedies are said to help balance the yin-yang mechanism in the system. Since ill health is often the symptom of a disturbed internal condition, the Orientalists treat it by correcting the cause and adjusting the yin-yang mechanism, thus easing the symptoms.

The wise Orientals were the first to realize the healing virtues of medicinal plants. They had a rich supply at their fingertips and they were able to survive throughout the centuries by using such all-natural medicinal plants. In our modern times, we are slowly recognizing the value of healing through Nature. Perhaps the "ancient" Orientals were more "modern" in their approach to healthful living than we care to admit.

How the Oriental Secret of Barley
Promotes Digestive Healing

Pearled barly (a cereal grass) has always been used by Oriental folk physicians for the healing and the rejuvenation of the digestive system. A simple, yet effective folk remedy was to make a barley brew that was to be sipped throughout the day while other foods were restricted or limited. This folk remedy has helped many people, even to this day.

How "Barley Brew" Soothed a
Housewife's Lifelong Indigestion

Housewife Selma D. was troubled with a burning sensation in her stomach; whenever she ate, she felt "gas bubbles" trapped within her digestive system. Often, she would feel the same "liquid burning," which went right up into her throat. It would give her a gagging sensation, causing her to choke and become nauseous. Selma D. tried many recommended treatments and drugs, which offered partial relief, but once the effects wore off, her sensitive stomach "screamed" whenever she ate a meal.

Selma was told of an Oriental folk healer who gave "digestive youth" to many who might otherwise have had perpetual stomach trouble. Accordingly, she prepared an all-natural barley brew as follows:

Boil one-quarter cup of all-natural pearled barley in two quarts of water. When the water has boiled down to about one quart, strain carefully. Drink this all-natural barley brew.

Feels Stomach Relaxation. Selma D. felt a general contentment and stomach relaxation. By the end of the day, she felt so soothed, she was eager to start eating the next day to see if this Oriental folk healer could make her enjoy digestion. Indeed, the next day, she was able to eat with much comfort and little distress. Selma D. decided to devote one day a week to a barley-brew program. Within a month, she had a digestive rejuvenation that enabled her to eat and digest her food with the gusto of a youngster — thanks to the Oriental barley folk healer.

Barley's Secret Rejuvenation Benefit: The barley brew offers a two-way digestive rejuvenation benefit. It has a *demulcent* response, in which it soothes the burning digestive actions, and it has a *mucilagenous* response, in which it introduces a natural oily substance, which helps to protect the abraded mucous membrane of the digestive system. This twin digestive rejuvenation benefit also helps promote the soothing of what might otherwise be an "aged" digestive system. Once the digestive system is thus soothed and healed, it can promote better assimilation of foods. Thanks to the Oriental secret of barley, Selma D. is able to join the tens of thousands of reported persons who found this natural healer the key to digestive rejuvenation!

How a Herb-Fruit-Barley Healer Helped
Establish Youthful Regularity

John L. was a "laxative slave": He was embarrassed by irregularity. He was resigned to the fate of taking tablets, candy-flavored laxatives, fizzes, powders and chewing gums, because he had a stuffed feeling that could not be relieved by natural methods. How could he break the laxative habit? He had read of the Oriental "forever young" digestive systems and came across an ancient secret of youthful regularity.

Just a few all-natural ingredients and the Oriental folk physicians said that youthful regularity could be restored. Here is how they prescribed this herb-fruit-barley healer:

Boil one-quarter cup of all-natural pearled barley in two quarts of water. When the water has boiled down to about one quart, strain carefully. To this, add 2 sliced raw figs, 1/2 teaspoon cut licorice root (available from most herbal pharmacies), 2 tablespoons organic sun-dried raisins. Mix all together and boil about 5 minutes. Strain. Now eat the solid portion. Follow with slow sipping of the liquid portion. (NOTE: Oriental folk physicians have recommended that this herb-fruit-barley healer be taken in the morning, on an empty stomach.)

John L. tried this Oriental folk healer as directed. He experienced a relief from fullness the first morning. It took four mornings before he was able to benefit from the folk healer. Thereafter, he needed to take it only once a week. He had also given up commercial chemicalized laxatives. Soon, his digestive system felt alert and healthy. He was "regular" and enjoyed youthful health — thanks to a time-tested, ancient but surprisingly effective Oriental healer.

Secret Benefit: The colloidal character of the liquid promoted a digestive action that led to internal balance. The yin-yang principle was thus established and regularity could be achieved.

How Eating an Asiatic Barley Bun Helps Promote Digestive Youth

Many Asiatics look to the Barley Bun as a special "offering" to the gods because it gives them such a feeling of digestive well-being and youth. Here's how to make this Barley Bun:

Combine these all-natural and organic ingredients: 1-1/2 cups barley meal, 1/4 cup honey, 1/2 teaspoonful of cinnamon powder, 1/2 cup of whole wheat unbleached flour. Combine together and divide into small buns or cakes. Bake in the oven until done. For many Asiatics, a Barley Bun is a youth restorative snack to be taken after each meal.

Secret Benefit: Unsaturated fatty acids from the whole grain combine with the minerals of the honey and help create a soothing and gentle healing effect upon the digestive tract. In many Middle Eastern countries, this ancient but delicious "folk healer" is used as an after dinner "snack" that tastes good and helps bring contentment to the digestive system.

The Secret Internal Cleansing Action of the Apple

While our modern world is familiar with the "apple a day keeps the doctor away" slogan, the ancient Orientals have long been familiar with the cleansing actions of the apple.

Among many Asiatic folk physicians, an apple was prescribed

when a person felt a weakened digestive system. The ancient Persian folk healers had this digestive folk remedy:

Persian Stomach Tonic

Shred an apple until it takes on the consistency of applesauce. Add one tablespoon honey. Sprinkle with sesame seeds. Eat with a spoon *before* beginning a meal — as an appetizer.

Secret Benefit: Royal physicians appointed to the ancient Persian courts would suggest this Persian stomach tonic *before* a meal as a means of stimulating sluggish digestive juices (enzymes) so that they could gush forth and thereby facilitate assimilation of food for healthful results.

How an Ancient "Apple Medicine" Helped Heal a Schoolteacher's Stomach Spasms

Schoolteacher Edith T. was the victim of years of stomach spasms. She described them as "butterflies" that torturously flickered around throughout the day or whenever she faced an unusual stress situation. True, she did face many schoolroom tensions that reacted on her digestive system, but the many antacids and the antispasmodics she took were of minimal value. She was always the victim of "knots" that tied her stomach up until she was almost doubled over with pain. Someone suggested she try to use an ancient folk remedy she had come across during a trade fair that featured Oriental exhibits and artifacts. This particular Oriental folk program was said to create an all-natural digestive aid that rivaled that of the modern synthetic medication.

The All-Natural Apple Medicine to Soothe a "Knotted Stomach"

Slice a whole apple. An organic apple is suggested since the rind and inner portions must be free of chemical sprays or preservatives. Gently pound the apple until it becomes slightly mashed. Sprinkle with cinnamon or honey, if desired. Now, eat the entire mashed apple, except for the stem and seeds. *Chew* very thoroughly before swallowing.

Suggestion: Oriental healers would suggest eating several of these "Apple Medicines" throughout the day, *between* meals, to enable its medicines to perform their healing functions.

Schoolteacher Obtains Relief
from Twisted Stomach Pains

Edith T. followed this simple, yet remarkably effective program daily. Within five days, her stomach pains subsided; the "butterflies" were gone and her entire digestive system felt young and healthy. She was relaxed, relieved, rejuvenated! All this, thanks to a simple plant healer from the Orient.

Secret Apple Rejuvenation Benefit: The all-natural medicinal substance in the mashed apple is *pectin*. This same therapeutic ingredient is manufactured by artifical means and is often upsetting to the already abused stomach.

The Orientals offered insight into the working of pectin. This all-natural medicine is found in the dilute acid extract of the inner portion of the rinds, and from the pomace (the natural medicinal portion of apples crushed by grinding). The pectin works to create a protective coating action by virtue of its benefit as an absorbent and demulcent; it also helps in soothing frazzled digestive nerves by supplying what we today call "galacturonic acid," which sucks up noxious substances and aids in their release. It is this self-cleansing action which promotes internal washing and a subsequent feeling of digestive youth.

Despite their ignorance of our modern scientific terms, the Orientals knew that a certain plant promoted healing and rejuvenation, and this was sufficient for them to prescribe it for treatments.

How a Lemon Helps Heal Throat Disorders

Folk healers among the people of Darjeeling and the Sikkim Himalayas, reportedly prescribed this simple program to help heal throat disorders such as catarrh, choking sensation, itching or sensitivities:

Slowly roast a ripe unpeeled lemon until it begins to crack open. Then take one teaspoonful of the juice with a little honey about once every hour. *Or,* take the same juice of the roasted lemon in a glass of boiled water. Flavor with honey. Sip slowly.

How to Use a Lemon to Heal Foot Disorders

The Orientals have always been great travelers; therefore, they have often been the victims of foot disorders. The writings of Marco Polo refer to these Mongolian-Manchurian, doctor-prescribed foot remedies that use the lemon:

How to Soothe Burning Soles and Heels

Rub sliced lemon over the entire burning soles and heels of the feet. The benefit here is that much toxin elimination takes place through the pores of the feet. Lemon applications facilitate such elimination and help disinfect against bacteria.

Foot Relaxation Lemon Rub: Caravan travelers would often soak their feet in comfortably hot water and follow with a thorough rubbing of the feet with lemon juice. The benefit here is in the contrasting actions of the hot water (opens the pores) and the lemon juice (presents a cooling, astringent action). This treatment is also said to promote healthy sleep, owing to its relaxing action on the foot nerves.

Natural Foot-Corn Remedy: In the writings of folk physicians of the Ceylon-India region, it was reported that when natives were troubled with "foot felons" (interpreted as corns or callouses), they follow this natural program: tie a fresh slice of lemon over the painful area and let it remain overnight. Repeat nightly until the growth or "felon" has gone.

How a Potato Helped Rejuvenate an Oriental Princess

It is recorded in the secret book of plant remedies, *Book of Songs (Shih Ching),* written by Manchurian folk physicians some 4,000 years ago, that a princess was worried about her aging appearance. Without offending the princess by referring to her age, the folk physicians simply prescribed the use of raw potatoes.

A few raw potatoes were shredded. The liquid pulp was to be used as a poultice against the face, or on other portions of the body that had wrinkles or blemishes. The princess followed the folk physicians' prescription, rubbed this juicy potato pulp over her skin at night. It is reported that just one week of this plant treatment helped "melt" her wrinkles, banish her age spots and clear her skin. She became the envy of the younger members of the Imperial Court.

Secret Benefit: The enzymes in raw potato pulp, combined with the Vitamin C and the natural starch, helped create a "skin food" that reportedly nourished the "starved" cellular tissues of the skin. Furthermore, the alkaline juices of the potato promoted an antiseptic action that gave a glowing look of youth. Much of the decaying skin was sloughed off by the acid portion of the pulp. Altogether, the princess was reportedly rejuvenated. The folk physicians were handsomely rewarded; their achievements were recorded in the secret *Book of Songs,* and it was up to their successors to slowly reveal the secrets to others in the Orient — and now in the West.

A Japanese Plant Healer for Poor Digestion

A comparatively recent Oriental digestive aid was revealed through Japanese writings, and through research in the areas of folk medicine. The Japanese folk doctors of a century ago prescribed the eating of raw radishes (including the green tops) as a means of helping to promote youthful digestion and a feeling of stomach contentment. It is believed that the rich vitamins, minerals and enzymes can serve to soothe and heal the flurries in the digestive system.

This all-natural medicinal healer was unearthed in a long-forgotten ship's log. A cargo ship made its way across the Pacific, laden with fresh raw fruits and vegetables. In the midst of the journey, several of the Japanese sailors developed severe stomach pains; the Captain was stricken, too. Someone remembered that one of his revered ancestors had praised radishes, with their green tops, as a divine palliative to painful stomach ache. Several of the stricken Japanese sailors, as well as the Captain, munched on the radishes from the ship's cargo. They experienced merciful relief. In this manner, an ancient Japanese folk healer contributed to modern medical knowledge.

How an Everyday Plant Helps Cleanse the Kidneys and Bladder

In the year 1556, it was announced that there were vacancies in the Imperial Academy of Medicine in Peking. Examinations were held, in which folk healers or recognized physicians could submit "divine remedies" that would help promote youth *from within.* These "primitive" Orientals realized that rejuvenation came from the internal being; hence, their request for such remedies.

One of the applicants, the noted Li Shih-chen (1518-1593), was said to "have no equal south of the Great Bear" (referring to the celestial sign) and was gifted in the knowledge of the "secrets of youth from within the body." Li Shih-chen was a physician who knew anatomy. He said that the key to youthful digestion was in having cleansed kidneys and youthful bladder function.

Carrot Prescription

Li Shih-chen offered this prescription, which he believed would help rejuvenate the kidneys, bladder and "adjoining parts":

Chop and dice raw carrots; use the carrot tops in the same chopped and diced form. Place in a kettle, fill with water, bring to a boil. Let stand until cool. Sip a "goodly portion" before each of your three daily meals. This folk medicine is said to put vital energy into the kidneys and bladder as well as connecting organs.

Reported Results: In his classic book written years later, entitled *The Network of Nerves and Vessels,* Li Shih-chen said that Peking royalists felt "reborn" with "young" digestion, and they immediately awarded him the coveted medical post in the Academy. Thus began his lifelong devotion to folk medicines. His book explains that certain ingredients (today identified as vitamins and minerals) are liberated through the boiling of the carrots and provide an "immediate remedial and youthful joy" to the kidneys and bladder.

The carrot is an everyday plant, but to the Orientals, it became a "youth food" for their digestive organs!

How Berries Act as an All-Natural Digestive Purification Tonic

Barbara G. thought that her poor digestion and pasty complexion were due to her long work-day indoors as a statistical typist. She shrugged off a health-minded friend's suggestion that a poor assimilative system means premature aging. But when her energy depleted, when her hands and feet felt cold, and when she felt "sour stomach" whenever she ate, she decided that improved digestion could perhaps, be the key to perpetual youth.

The Cantonese Purification Tonic

Reading about the Orient after China was admitted to the United Nations, Barbara G. came across an item of interest. It said that Cantonese folk physicians often prescribed raw blueberries as a means of boosting a sluggish digestive system to bring the "bloom of roses" to one's cheeks. She tried this reported *Digestive Purification Tonic:*

In a bowl, mash a portion of raw blueberries. Add honey to taste. Eat with a spoon.

Feels Partial Relief: Barbara G. felt some relief. Her digestive powers improved and she felt a bit lighter and more energetic. Thus encouraged, she followed the next folk medicine:

Blueberry Leaf Tea: From a herbalist, she obtained blueberry leaves. At home, she steeped one tablespoon of the cut, dried leaves in a cup of hot water and flavored it with honey. Barbara G. followed the Cantonese folk doctor's prescription to drink one such cup, four times a day.

Results: After seven days of this folk medicine, she felt more alert, more youthful, her skin took on the glow of youth, and she walked with a sprightly step. Barbara G. felt alive, alert and good all over, thanks to the Cantonese berry program.

Secret Blueberry Healing Benefit: The Cantonese folk doctors were aware that the leaves of the blueberry possessed medicinal benefits. Our scientists agree that the steamed blueberry leaves release a substance called *myrtillin,* which perks up sluggish digestion, heals stomach unrest and helps create a form of blood purification.

The blueberries themselves contain calcium, phosphorus and iron, as well as manganese. The manganese, which is released through mashing of the blueberries, works as a catalyst within the digestive circulation; that is, it helps send valuable enzymes and minerals into the bloodstream. This creates a purification that is rejuvenating and helps enhance the workings of the digestive organs. Blueberries — a time-tested Cantonese folk medicine to help promote youthful digestion via a healthful plant.

The Tibetan Clove Cocktail Youth Secret

Many explorers throughout the centuries have come home from brief visits to forbidden Tibet, the magical-mysterious land that is considered the roof of the world, and all have expressed amazement at the perpetual youth of the Tibetan people, especially the holy lamas (priests). These sacred men often reach well beyond the century mark in age, often nearing a century and a half of productive and youthful life.

From fragments of writings, some secrets have been revealed that may be the source of the Tibetan "forever youthful" appearance. One such secret is that of the clove cocktail, as we call it today. Here's how it is made:

Clove Cocktail Recipe from Tibet: Use a whole and unground organic clove. Select about 4 such clove buds. Let steep in a cup of boiled water up to 5 minutes. Strain. Sip slowly.

Youth Benefits: Ingredients in this ancient herb act as a stimulating carminative to promote overall assimilation. It is believed to help stimulate a sluggish circulation and thereby promote youthful digestion and metabolism.

The "secret" was revealed through caravan merchants from the Molucca Islands and Zanzibar, which are the chief sources of the clove plant. The merchants were paid handsomely for regular shipments of cloves through India and up the steep mountain trails of the Himalayas. They bribed lesser officials of the Tibetan monasteries, learned of the secret, and recorded it in various scrolls and records.

The Orientals have long felt that the benefits from cloves can be healthful to the digestive and internal organs. It worked for the Tibetans, and it should be helpful to our modern health and youth seekers.

For almost fifty centuries, everyday plants have been used as medicinal healings for the digestive system, helping to build and rebuild youth. Today, more and more, we are understanding the relationship between all-natural medicines and coveted youth. Throughout the many centuries, the Orientals have held the belief that perpetual youth begins with healthy digestion. This is part of the principle of maintaining the proper balance of yin and yang elements. Use plants for healing; enjoy the rewards of youth.

The Orientals note that everything in the universe is interrelated, and that man is part of Nature. For this reason, youth comes from Nature. Thus, they have been able to restore harmony and thereby prolong digestive youth with plants; nature has shown them the way. Let Nature show you the way to digestive youth, too.

HIGHLIGHTS:

1. Secret Oriental books of rejuvenation place emphasis upon the use of plants for healing. Correct the digestion and enjoy extended youth.
2. Barley is a plant food that helps relax, refresh, and rejuvenate the digestive system. Various barley brews and tonics gave Selma D. a "young stomach" and a forever-young lease on life.
3. A simple herb-fruit-barley healer freed John L. from the use of laxatives and made him feel young all over.
4. Asiatics have used a Persian stomach tonic to bolster a tired digestive system.
5. An ancient Oriental apple medicine helped heal a schoolteacher's stomach spasms.
6. Folk healers from Darjeeling and the Sikkim Himalayas have reported that the use of a lemon can help stimulate an overall feeling of well-being.
7. A potato reportedly rejuvenated a Manchurian princess and helped her roll back the years.
8. A locally available plant is looked upon by the Japanese as a means of promoting youthful digestion.
9. Rejuvenate the kidneys and bladder with Li Shih-chen's special plant prescription, made right in your own kitchen.
10. Self-purification, as practiced by the Cantonese, helped Barbara G. relax and rejuvenate her digestive system.
11. A simple clove cocktail is revered as a Tibetan youth secret. Make it in your own home for just a small cost. All products are available at most herbal pharmacies, health stores or local supermarkets.

5

How a Controlled Oriental Rice Diet Helps Regulate Blood Pressure the Natural Way

An ancient Oriental food is the basis for modern healing of problems involving high blood pressure, hypertension and nervous unrest. As a much-revered Oriental food, rice has always been considered a magical healer in the East. One of the earliest mentions of rice dates back to ca. 2800 B.C., when a Chinese emperor established a ceremonial ordinance for the planting of rice that would later be used by the royal physicians for healing purposes.

Rice was originally believed to have medicinal values that could restore tranquility and peace to the easily upset members of the royal court. The folk physicians would also prescribe a rice fast to ailing Orientals as a means of helping to re-establish the disturbed yin-yang balance. In many early Oriental writings, it is said that natural, whole-grain brown rice is a "perfect" healing food because it is so delicately balanced by Nature. (Macrobiotic physicians corroborate this finding by calling natural brown rice the perfect yin-yang balanced food.)

From fragmented writings that have come down to us throughout the centuries, it is mentioned that rice was being grown back in 3000 B.C., when it appeared as a plant called "Newaree" in ancient India. The holy healers would prescribe rice to those who were said to be possessed of demons, which was an emotional way of saying that the persons were nervous, or victims of hypertension. Many of the Indian holy healers would urge their followers to abstain from most foods and subsist on brown rice for a few days as a means of helping to create a balanced condition, which would promote better health.

Rice is Revered as a Food of Divine Health

Some of the earliest manuscripts of India contain descriptions of rice being used in religious offerings. The ancients revered this grain as a food of divine health. Similar evidences of the importance of rice as a source of health have been found in the early literature of Thailand, Burma, Malaya and Indochina. The Orientals have always held rice in veneration, recognizing that it could promote a feeling of well-being and youthful health. To this day, rice is considered a creation of a gracious Deity and a source of divine health for mortals. (In some modern cultures, rice is even showered upon newly married couples as a symbol of the marriage's long life.)

Basic Health Benefits of Rice

The health benefits of rice have been explored by modern scientists. They have confirmed what the ancient Oriental folk physicians have long maintained: that the eating of brown rice is a source of serenity and tranquility and a divine source of all the elements needed to help create better health. As interpreted by modern scientists, here is what rice will do for your health:

Rice is a Prime Source of Meatless Protein

Those who are concerned about the blood-stimulating properties of meat would do well to consider a meatless source of protein. Rice protein, which comprises up to 8% of the grain, has a special benefit: *rice protein has eight of the essential amino acids (out of about eleven) in a delicately balanced yin-yang proportion.* When rice protein is metabolized into health-building amino acids, a complete internal rejuvenation takes place. These rice-created amino acids build resilient muscles, healthy skin and hair and clearer eyesight. Amino acids will then enter into the blood and lymph to nourish the heart and lungs, tendons and ligaments, brain, nervous system and glandular network. Rice offers these delicately balanced amino acids to the system as a means of helping to build health.

Vitamins Help Create Youthful Vitality. Natural brown rice is a prime source of the healthy B-complex vitamins.   In particular, rice offers thiamine, riboflavin and niacin, which are needed to promote youthful energy and to nourish the skin and blood vessels. Many nervous, tense people are in need of the soothing B-complex vitamins found in natural brown rice.

Minerals Offer Magic Youthfulness. An abundance of minerals in natural brown rice help to nourish the hormonal system (secret of magic youthfulness), heal wounds, create a healthy heartbeat and regulate blood pressure. In particular, rice has a high amount of calcium, which soothes and relaxes the nervous system and helps calm symptoms of hypertension. Furthermore, rice releases iron to enrich the bloodstream, and offers phosphorus and potassium to work with other nutrients and maintain internal water balance. This is a principle of the yin-yang balance. The nutrients all converge to help correct disturbances and bring about order and harmony from within. This is the greatly desired Oriental secret of good health. Rice serves as the "divine source" of restoring internal harmony. In our modern times, we know that this restoration of balance is needed to help soothe problems of hypertension and related nervous disorders.

Rice is Easily Digested. Rice, which is about 98% digestible, is one of the most easily and quickly digested of all foods, being fully digested in one hour, while meats may require up to four hours. Also, rice starch is different from other grain starches because it is 100% amylopectin — the most rapidly and completely digested grain starch. This makes it an ideal health food for those who seek speedy, healthy assimilation.

Rice Has Low Fiber Content. Rice has a very low fiber content, making it extremely soothing to the digestive system. Many folks who have problems such as colitis, ulcers, internal upheaval, hypertension and heart unrest, will welcome the soothing low fiber content of natural brown rice.

Rice is Low-Fat, Low-Cholesterol, Low-Salt. These three benefits are especially welcomed by the hypertensive person. Rice contains a tiny trace of fat (a grain fat, which is considered less harmful than meat fat), and it is also very low in cholesterol. Rice is virtually free of sodium or salt, making it an Oriental "perfect" food for those hypertensive people who are on salt-restricted diets.

Rice Offers More Benefits. Modern researchers have probed for the secret of the relative absence of hypertension, high blood pressure and heart distress in Oriental countries. They have noted that wherever rice is used as the main food, there is a corresponding benefit of youthful vitality and a very low rate of the problems of hypertension, which often plague other cultures. The reason is also attributed to the Orientals less frequent use of meat products as sources of protein. This helps create a more tranquil balance of the delicate blood pressure mechanisms.

Dr. Walter Kempner, of Duke University, made a 20-year study of rice-eating nations and reported that a special diet, followed in conjunction with advice from your family physician, is helpful in soothing high blood pressure and is a healing aid for related cardiac and kidney disorders. Orientals have shown a remarkable resistance to these disorders and it is believed that dependence upon rice as a meatless source of nutrients may be the secret of their youthful health. Today, throughout the Orient, many health resorts have combined the ancient "sacred food" of rice with modern discoveries and come up with various programs that have reportedly helped create a beneficial yin-yang balance and subsequent relief of hypertension.

The Favored Health-Building Rice of the Orient

The ancient and modern Oriental folk healers have always used *natural brown rice* as a key to youthful health-building. In our modern times, we have seen the emergence of bleached and processed milled white rice. This is shunned by the Orientals. The processing removes many of the valuable B-complex vitamins and some of the minerals, too. Furthermore, chemical residues used in processing often cling to the polished white particles, and this is considered harmful to one's health by modern folk physicians.

In selecting rice, choose *natural brown rice*. It is available at almost any health food store or supermarket. This gives you the whole unpolished grain of rice — a prime source of nutrients. It has a delightful, nut-like flavor and chewy texture, and it lends itself well to just about any meal.

Two Varieties of Rice

1. Long-Grain Rice. The grain of long-grain rice is four times as long as it is wide. When cooked, the grains tend to separate and become light and fluffy. It is especially good for salads, curries, stews, chicken or meat dishes, or as a side dish with a sauce or gravy. This rice is also excellent for casseroles and combination dishes.

2. Short and Medium Grain Rice. These varieties have short, plump grains, which cook tender and moist, with the particles tending to cling together. They are favored by many and are especially good for croquettes, puddings or rice rings, which require a tender rice that is easily molded.

The Oriental Way to Healthy Rice Cooking

The modern Orientals have taken this ancient, healthy food and created ways to cook it with good health in mind. Here are some of the most popular methods:

The Fluffy-Rice Method: Measure 1 cup uncooked natural brown rice into a 3-quart saucepan with a tightly fitted lid. Add 2 cups water. Heat to boiling, stirring once or twice. Reduce heat to simmer. Cover and cook 14 minutes *without removing lid or stirring*. All water should be absorbed. Test the rice by tasting it to see that it is tender. Simmer a little longer if needed. Remove from heat. Turn rice into serving dish. Fluff with fork or slotted spoon.

The Oven-Bake Method: Heat oven to 350°F. Combine 1 cup uncooked natural brown rice with 2 cups water into a 3-quart baking dish. Cover. Bake 25 or 30 minutes or until rice is tender.

The Feathered-Rice Method: Heat oven to 375°F. Spread 1 cup natural brown rice in a shallow baking pan. Bake, stirring occasionally, until rice grains are golden brown. Remove pan from the oven. Now turn oven heat to 400°F. Put toasted rice into 1-1/2-quart casserole with a tightly fitting cover. Stir in 2-1/2 cups boiling water. Cover. Bake 20 minutes. (NOTE: You can toast a quantity of rice at one time, then store it in a tightly covered jar for future use.)

The Double-Boiler Method: Many Orientals cook rice in milk. A modern method is to cook over boiling water; that is, in the top of a double boiler. Place 1 cup natural brown rice in the top of a double boiler with 3-1/2 cups of milk. Heat to boiling, then place over boiling water and cook, covered, for 40 minutes, or until milk is absorbed.

Oriental Secret of Rice Cookery: Simple — use 2 cups of water with each 1 cup of natural brown rice. That's all there is to it!

The enviable serenity and well-balanced blood pressure as well as youthful health of the Orientals may well be due to their judicious use of natural brown rice in special programs as prescribed by past and present folk physicians.

Ten Secret Oriental Rice Fasting Programs and How They Help Balance Blood Pressure and Promote Youthful Health

Ancient Oriental folk physicians reported that when "divine rice" was eaten, there was a "divine reward" of prosperously good health. (This points out that various health problems did exist in the ancient Orient, probably due to the Oriental's affinity for strong spices and seasoned foods.) It is reasonable to interpret the Oriental rice fasting program as being a low-salt or no-salt program, and this is the first step in helping to correct imbalanced blood pressure. The next step is to combine rice with specific foods to create a soothing harmony.

The yin-yang principle is manifest throughout these Oriental rice fasting programs, which have been interpreted in the light of modern knowledge of nutritional therapies. Many of these rice fasting programs have been used by Orientals as well as by visitors to Oriental countries at exclusive health resorts and plush rejuvenation retreats, and they may be followed in your own home with a minimum of effort.

Before You Begin: Follow the Oriental rice fasting program in the comfort of your home. Your mind and body should be relaxed. Try to free yourself from any tension-causing situations, since these may upset the internal harmony created by re-establishment of the yin-yang balance. A soothing environment is most helpful when following the fast.

Length of Fast: Oriental folk physicians of the past and present have often noted soothing results in patients who adhered to the rice fast for three to five days. Since each individual is different, be guided by your own awareness of natural healing as you progress.

Use Organic Foods: All foods used should be of an organic, all-natural, chemical-free source. Modern Oriental folk physicians explain that chemicals or harsh and volatile additives in foods disrupt the harmony of the body. As an example, they point to the health of the ancients who used organic foods for healing. Today, organic foods are again available through special food outlets and health food shoppes. You would do well to use them exclusively in order to help cleanse and rebuild your body.

Rice Fasting Programs are Interchangeable: Many of the modern health resorts suggest using interchangeable rice fasting programs. You may follow one program one day, then another the next day. Modern Oriental folk physicians report more success if only *one* rice fast is followed throughout the day, however. They frown upon dividing the day into different rice fasts. Select your desired rice fasting program for the day. Change to another one the next day, if you wish. This helps offer a variety of taste.

Now, let's glimpse into the past and see how traditional rice fasting programs can be "Nature's tranquilizers" in light of the modern scientific understanding of nutrition.

Oriental Secret #1 —
Rice-With-Fruit Fasting Program

Throughout the day, eat natural brown rice with a wide assortment of seasonal *raw* fruits. With each of your meals, have a large bowl of natural brown rice and a selection of different fresh fruits. You may combine the raw fruits in the same bowl with the rice, but the fruits *must* be raw. Chew thoroughly.

Health Benefit: Enzymes in the raw fruits work upon the vitamins, minerals and protein in the rice to create a skillful blending of nutrients that promote cleansing of the bloodstream. The presence of this mixture enables the metabolism to take the protein's nitrogen, sulfur and phosphorus and transform these substances into natural tranquilizers in the system. This balance facilitates cellular metabolism and promotes "body neutrality," or a balanced yin-yang harmony, which is the key to regulated blood pressure.

How an Overworked Office Worker Benefited from the Rice-With-Fruit Fasting Program: Overworked and overwrought, Viola H. had a history of high blood pressure. Her skin was blotchy. She had recurring headaches in the region of her temples (a common hypertensive reaction) and was so nervous that slight noises would drive her up the wall. No doubt, she was overworked. She sought a natural health program and selected the rice-with-fruit fasting program. Just four days and her heart poundings eased, her skin cleared up, her headaches were less severe, although mildly recurring. She felt more relaxed and minor noises did not make her shriek and rant. It was a natural program that helped re-establish her body harmony and now Viola H. was able to enjoy better life, do a better job, and have a more relaxed healthful life.

Oriental Secret #2 —
Rice-With-Fruit Juice Fasting Program

Throughout the day, use natural brown rice as your only solid food. Cook it in any manner, but *do not use any salt.* With each of your meals, drink freshly prepared natural raw fruit juices. Beverages should be comfortably cool and *not* ice cold.

Health Benefit: Amino acid molecules in the digested rice combine with the valuable and natural fruit sugar, fructose. In digestive metabolic combination, the nutrients are formed into malic acid, citric acid and glycogen. This is stored within the body so that it may be used to produce energy when required. This spares the body the need to drain out much of its reserves during stress-tension situations and does much to promote natural tranquility. The availability of metabolized glucose is a known factor in helping to keep down excessive cholesterol as well as in promoting better relaxation. The natural carbohydrates of rice join with the natural sugars of freshly prepared fruit juices to create this speedy source of healthy vitality. Raw juices are preferable, according to Oriental folk medicine, because they require less digestive effort and are speedily available for "instant vitality."

How an Engineer Meets the Demands of his Job: Whenever Phillip F. is faced with the deadlines and overtime tensions of his engineering profession, he prepares for the stress and hypertension with this rice and fruit juice fasting program. He reports that if he starts the program one day before his anticipated heavy work, and continues throughout the work schedule on the fasting, he has a clearer head and feels more relaxed, light and healthy. Once the tension situation is over, he goes back to his usual living methods. He calls the Oriental secret his "natural pep program."

Oriental Secret #3 —
Rice-With-Vegetables Fasting Program

Throughout the day, eat natural brown rice with a wide assortment of seasonal *raw* vegetables. You may combine the raw vegetables in the same bowl with the rice, but the vegetables *must* be raw. Chew thoroughly.

The Unique Health Benefit of Rice Protein: The protein in rice has a unique way of enhancing the protein in raw vegetables. The sulfur and isoleucine of rice take the protein from raw vegetables, give them an energizing effect and blend together during the metabolic process. This creates a youthful regeneration from within and a source of vital energy. The secret here is to eat the assorted vegetables *at the same time,* so that the amino acids in one vegetable are joined with the amino acids offered by the others. Together, they are gathered up by the nutrients in the rice so they can be used by the electrolytic processes to build a source of energy within the body. This supplements any deficiencies that might otherwise cause nervous high-strung symptoms.

How a Salesman Achieved Muscular Relaxation: Hypertensive situations caused Charles Y. to experience muscle knots and tense constrictions throughout the back of his neck and shoulders. He had always envied a certain Oriental importer's serenity in the midst of sales deadlines, and one day he learned the secret. Charles Y. tried a three-day rice-with-vegetables program. He experienced relief when his knotted muscles "melted" and his muscular constriction loosened up. Because he was always traveling about, he found it difficult to maintain such a program; so he went on a simple fasting program as regularly as possible and at least enjoyed partial benefits.

Oriental Secret #4 —
Rice-With-Vegetable Juice Fasting Program

Throughout the day, use natural brown rice as your only solid food. Cook it in any manner, but *do not use any salt.* With each of your meals, drink freshly prepared, natural raw vegetable juices. Beverages should be comfortably cool and *not* ice cold.

Health Benefit: The rice, with its high satiety value and low sodium content, blends with the fresh mineral taste of raw juices. In particular, rice protein provides a spark-plug to the precious enzymes in the raw juices. The green leaves of the vegetables, when squeezed, provide speedily assimilated vitamins and nutrients that are taken up by the rice proteins to create an alkaline reaction in the body. This helps create a more favorable acid-alkaline balance (principle of the sacred yin-yang harmony) and promotes soothing relaxation. The easily assimilable protein of the rice works upon the readily available raw enzymes and nutrients of the vegetable juices. This works to improve regularity, build resistance to ailments, boost the regularity of the heart rhythm and stabilize the blood pressure. It is the combination of these factors that is the basis for this Oriental health secret.

How a Librarian Became Relaxed, Refreshed — and Younger-Looking: Maryann W. looked much older than her middle 40's. Long indoor hours, laboring over filing cabinets and straightening book stacks, did take their toll. She felt nervous — "fit to be tied." Her face was pale, her features drooped; she slumped in her seat. She looked decades older!

It was a returnee from a Hawaiian health spa who insisted Maryann try this simple fast. It was said to be an ancient Oriental rejuvenation program. Scoffing, Maryann W. tried a rice and vegetable juice program for two days. From the start, she felt a "lifting of weight" from her shoulders. It took four days before her face was alertly pink, her nerves were calm, and she walked and worked with the agility of youth. She had used an Oriental all-natural program to restore her upset yin-yang balance and, as a result, she radiated good health.

Oriental Secret #5 —
Rice-With-Milk Fasting Program

Throughout the day, use natural brown rice as your only solid food. Cook it in any manner, but *do not use any salt.* With each of your meals, drink fresh milk. It should be comfortably cool and *not* ice cold.

Health Benefit: The nutrients in the rice form a unique balance with those in the milk. In particular, milk has notable amino acid strengths in isoleucine and lysine. These two amino acids are further strengthened by rice protein and are able to form stronger body-building blocks. The natural lactic acid of milk will work with rice protein to aid in the absorption of iron. The combination of both rice and milk will actually *increase* iron absorption because the milk sugar is then converted into lactic acid by other available nutrients. This creates a marvelous body balance that glows with radiant internal health and external youth.

How an Accountant Uses a Rice-Milk Fast for Rejuvenation: Once a week, Donald I enjoys a simple rice-milk fast. As a certified accountant, he is subjected to continual tensions. Wanting to control his blood pressure and enjoy better health, he tries this one-day rice-milk fast at the *beginning* of his work week. He finds that it promotes internal vigor, his mind becomes youthfully alert, and he no longer makes errors in organizing his accounting systems. He rightfully says it is "like being born anew."

Oriental Secret #6 —
Rice-With-Legumes (Beans) Fasting Program

Throughout the day, eat natural brown rice with a variety of freshly cooked beans. (You may combine the cooked brown rice with the cooked beans.) Chew thoroughly.

Health Benefit: Almost all forms of legumes, such as beans, lentils, black beans, soybeans, garbanzos and baked beans, are at least 20% protein. This protein is taken by rice protein and metabolized into amino acids, which are then passed into the bloodstream to be carried throughout the body. This rice-metabolized bean protein works to help construct new body tissue and produce such youth-creating substances as anti-bodies, hormones, blood tissues and enzymes. This rice fasting program will give your body such amino acids (which cannot be made in the body) as tryptophane, lysine, methionine, phenylalanine, threonine, valine, leucine and isoleucine. These are all essential to health. The Orientals may not have known their technical names, but they were aware of their presence and health influences. Thus, they urged fasting on rice and beans so that these nutrients could be created, without the interference of other foods.

How Mona Rid Herself of Nervous Headaches and Blurred Vision: Mona M. could scarcely read the timetable charts in her work as an airline reservations clerk. She knew she had neglected herself by keeping late hours and being careless about her diet. With the threat of losing her job, she started remedial action. An Oriental traveler boasted about a health resort in the Pacific that used fasting for healing, so she decided to try the program. Mona M. went on a rice and bean fast. There was so much improvement that, in three days, her headaches were gone and her vision improved. The amino acids had "free play" within her body and, thus, caused a healing and rejuvenation process within her that she previously thought to be impossible.

**Oriental Secret #7 —
Rice-With-Seeds Fasting Program**

Throughout the day, eat natural brown rice with a variety of different raw seeds such as sunflower seeds, sesame seeds, millet, groats, etc. You may combine the cooked brown rice with the raw seeds. Chew especially thoroughly in this program.

Health Benefit: The protein in seeds combines very efficiently with the protein in rice. The natural vitamins and minerals blend together and work in harmony with the nutrients of seeds to promote better assimilation and youthful digestion. In particular Vitamin B1 is taken up by the rice and used to help soothe a frazzled nervous system. This vitamin is highly perishable and easily destroyed. But in the presence of rice protein, it is completely utilized. Rice protein appears to complement and enhance the nerve-strengthening powers of Vitamin B1 in the seeds, hence, their value in this simple combination.

How This Program Helps Restore Cheer and Youthful Alertness: In a reported health experiment, a group of persons were irritable, quarrelsome, forgetful, and suffered erratic blood pressure readings. They also had insomnia, suffered from heart palpitations, and had cold hands and feet. This group was then put on the special rice and seeds program in order to restore deficiencies. In due time, they were cheerful and youthfully alert. They reported feelings of unusual well-being and vitality as the remaining symptoms slowly subsided.

Reason? The Vitamin B1 helped make up for deficiencies. In the Orient, a combined rice and seeds program is prescribed by folk physicians for those who are perpetually tired, high-strung or disagreeable. The combination fasting program helps make up for deficiencies and restore good health of body and mind.

Oriental Secret #8 —
Rice-With-Seed Sprouts Fasting Program

Throughout the day, eat natural brown rice with prepared seed sprouts, which are sold at most health food stores. You may make your own sprouts by soaking clean organic seeds overnight in a wide-mouthed jar. In the morning, drain. (Save liquid for soups, broths or green drinks.) Place soaked seeds in the jar, cover the top with nylon tulle or stainless steel screen wire. Screw the lid on tightly. Water the seeds under the tap about three times a day. Turn it on its side in a bowl in order to drain. It takes up to two days to have a jar of healthful seed sprouts. Eat these with brown rice in one bowl, or separately. It is important to masticate this food thoroughly.

Health Benefit: Seed sprouting increases the precious B-complex and C vitamin potency. Furthermore, Vitamin E, as well as many enzymes, is increased. When these nutrients are combined with rice protein, the reaction within the system is to build an *enzyme,* or "magical nutrient," which actually makes cells younger. Seed sprouts become the easiest protein to be digested. It is the complementary action of one nutrient upon the other in this fasting secret that makes it a source of youth. The Orientalists knew that the *combination* worked youth wonders. Many kept these formulae in secret, but many others shared the knowledge so that future generations could reap their benefits.

Self-Renewal Fasting Program: Although Elliot N. cannot watch his diet too carefully because he is a field surveyor and is constantly on the road, he uses a rice-and-seed sprout fasting program, one day a week, to "self-renew" and to "self-recharge" his worn out cells and, thus, to enjoy a feeling of renewed youth. Elliot claims that this Oriental fasting secret keeps him cool, calm and collected, and that it serves to reduce the symptoms of work-induced hypertension.

Oriental Secret #9 — Rice-With-Brewer's Yeast Fasting Program

Throughout the day, eat natural brown rice to which small portions of brewer's yeast have been added. This is a food yeast that is sold at most health food shoppes and many corner supermarkets. It is an all-natural plant food that is a rich source of vitamins, minerals and proteins, too. Yeast has all the elements of the B-complex vitamin family; it also has 16 of the 20 amino acids. One tablespoon of yeast offers as much protein as 1/4 cup of wheat germ, as much calcium as 1/2 cup of orange juice, as much phosphorus as 1/4 pound of fillet of haddock, as much iron as 1 cup of cooked spinach — all this and much, much more. It was a well-known health food in ancient days, and it is popular throughout the Orient today.

Health Benefit: Rice carbohydrates and vitamins combine with the high-quality and highly concentrated protein in the yeast to create a synergetic reaction, which helps to build and rebuild the body organs and systems. In combination, a rice and yeast fast can create a "magic" rejuvenation benefit. In particular, this action sends a stream of biotin, a vitality-vitamin, into tired organs, thus promoting a youthful feeling of well-being.

Simple Program Soothes and Improves Health: Adelle O. had a hectic schedule — managing her busy household and then going to her part-time job. She needed a vacation, but because she was unable to go away, she followed an Oriental folk program of using this rice-and-yeast fast as an "internal vacation." Adelle O. devoted about one day a week to this time-tested folk program. She felt emotionally and physically rejuvenated and her blood pressure became more relaxed. Her usually lethargy feeling went away and she began to sleep better, too. Adelle O. found that this Oriental folk secret enabled her to cope with tensions and to think more clearly, and many others have reported similar benefits.

Oriental Secret # 10 — Rice-With-Fish Fasting Program

Throughout the day, eat natural brown rice with baked, boiled or broiled fish. Select fresh water or salt water fish, but in either case, it is preferable to use organic fish.

Health Benefit: Organic fish is an especially good food to combine with the nutrients offered by rice. Unlike animal meats, organic fish are not given chemical hormones and tranquilizers, nor are they fed on commercially fertilized soils covered with poison sprays. Thus, they should help to create better harmony in conjunction with the nutrients in organic rice.

Tip: Enhance your health with the high iodine content of salt water fish. (Fresh water fish may be lower or lacking in iodine.) The iodine in salt water fish blends with the carbohydrates and vitamins in the rice to create an unusually high lysine content, which helps boost internal health. Fish and rice are well-known for being staple foods in the Orient. Together, they can promote a harmonious balance in the diet.

How a Factory Foreman Controls Hypertensive Outbursts: Whenever factory foreman George Q. goes on a rice-and-fish fasting program he is able to control the temperamental outbursts which are often symptoms of his hypertension. (The nutrient complementarity helps soothe his circulatory system.) He is grateful for this Oriental secret, and his co-workers are glad when he is able to act and talk with calmness. One problem does exist: George likes heavily salted and seasoned foods; so his healing is of a temporary nature. But a little healing is better than none at all!

Controlled Fasting: The Healing Secret from the Orient

Innumerable folk physicians throughout the Orient, from hundreds of centuries ago right up to the present time, have recognized that controlled fasting (not a starvation diet) can be healing to the mind as well as to the body. The secret is that when natural brown rice is combined with *one* other food, these foods converge upon each other and issue forth nutrients that work in harmony There is no interference from other foods. The digestive-assimilation system can work unimpeded to help restore health, create Oriental-type serenity, and make life worth living again!

MAIN POINTS:

1. Natural brown rice was prescribed by Oriental folk physicians as a foundation for internal rejuvenation in a set of ten controlled fasting programs.
2. Select any one or more of the ten programs and do as the Orientals do, to begin your health restorative objective.
3. The ten described case histories are reported revelations of the benefits of Oriental fasting with rice and any of the ten listed foods.

6

The Forever-Young Health Secrets from the Long-Living Abkhasians

In a certain region of Eurasia, natives live to be 100 years of age, and even older in many cases. In addition to enjoying long lives, the natives are pictures of youthful health, enjoy freedom from the so-called ravages of civilization, and are known for remaining remarkably free from conditions of ill health. Since 1932, the "forever-young" health secrets of these people have been studied systematically by competent European investigators. Gradually, their health programs and practices have been released. Today, many are discovering that it is possible to live to be 100, or even older, without the infirmities of "old age," by following an all-natural program based upon this modern-day Shangri-La.

The Modern Land of Perpetual Youth and Health

This land is known as the Abkhasian Republic — one of the republics of the USSR. Abkhasia is a subtropical region on the coast along the Black Sea, alpine-like if you travel directly back from the sea; the region extends through the populated lowlands and valleys to the main range of the towering Caucasus Mountains.

The native Abkhasians draw from a rich heritage that has been vividly influenced by nearly 1,000 years of Asian culture. In the past, Orientals from the Near East and the Far East had occupied their land, bringing Asian influences that included the Sunni sect of Islam, primitive animal sacrifices at family shrines, and folk medicine secrets of healing. Asian influences have survived into the 20th Century, and the health secrets have enabled the Abkhasians to enjoy perpetual youth and health.

Longevity is the Rule, Rather Than the Exception

Researchers who have investigated the health secrets of the Abkhasians report that longevity is an accepted rule, rather than an exception. A lifespan that extends up to 120 years of youthful vitality is quite common.

In one small village of 1200 people, there were 71 men and 110 women between 81 and 90; there were 19 people over the age of 91, and all were healthy and capable of taking care of themselves.

Vitality at Advanced Age

In a reported investigation, it was explained that 4 out of every 10 Abkhasians over the age of 90 enjoy vision youthful enough to be able to read or thread a needle without eyeglasses. Furthermore, 4 out of every 10 Abkhasians over the age of 90 had reasonably good hearing. A close study indicated that there were no reported cases of senility or emotional decline in the many Abkhasians who were over 100. These Asian-influenced people were clear and logical in their thoughts. They were physically alert, neat and clean, and they indicated a healthy interest in family and social affairs.

Health Secrets are All-Natural

The long-living Abkhasians use all-natural living programs in order to enjoy youthful health. They use no synthetics, artificial stimulants or chemical influences. Instead, they rely upon simple, all-natural programs that have become their health secrets for long and vitality-blessed lives. So natural is it for the Abkhasians to live long, that they just do not have any phrase for "old people." Those who pass the age of 100 are referred to as "long-living people." They have learned how to maintain a healthful internal balance based upon their Eurasian and Oriental influences from past centuries and have, as a result, reaped the rewards of all-natural living.

Ten Health Secrets of the Abkhasians

Here are the reported ten health secrets of these forever-young Eurasian peoples:

1. **All food is to be eaten slowly.** The Abkhasians eat leisurely and with comfort; there is no rush. All food is cut into small pieces and served on platters. Abkhasians take small bites of food and chew very slowly.

Secret Benefit: Slow and careful chewing stimulates the enzymatic flow of ptyalin and maltase, creating healthful digestion of the carbohydrates. This leads to better assimilation of youth-building nutrients.

2. **All foods are prepared and eaten at the meal. No leftovers are ever used.** A probable Oriental folk prescription is now part of Abkhasian daily living; namely, all food that is cooked should be eaten at the ensuing meal. No leftovers are ever used; most Abkhasians shun day-old food as being unhealthy.

Secret Benefit: Leftover foods are often depleted or void of valuable nutrients; they are often indigestible, interfere with assimilation of other nutrients and become "empty foods" that offer bulk and little else.

3. **Meat is eaten once or twice weekly and must be freshly killed.** The Abkhasians prefer chicken and beef. They require their meat only once or twice weekly and insist that it be freshly slaughtered. The two customary cooking methods are either broiling or boiling and, in either case, only to the absolute minimum.

Secret Benefit: The high vitamin, mineral and protein content of meat is enhanced if freshly prepared by either broiling or boiling. These two processes make the meat easier to digest and nutrients are able to create internal rejuvenation when transformed into amino acids through the assimilative process.

4. **A healthful bread substitute is salt-free corn meal mash.** Called *abista,* this is prepared by using corn meal mash cooked in water, without any salt. Abkhasian corn meal is whole grain. They use it as we use bread, except that it is always eaten warm.

Secret Benefit: Organic or whole-grain corn meal contains the valuable germ which includes the precious B-complex, youth-building Vitamin E and many minerals and enzymes. Corn meal is also a prime source of potassium, a mineral which helps to promote healthy heart functioning.

5. **Dairy products eaten daily are cheese (also homemade goat milk cheese) and two glasses of buttermilk.** It is customary for the healthy Abkhasians to eat cheese daily and to consume at least two glasses of buttermilk each day.

Secret Benefit: The unpasteurized milk in dairy products comes from cows that are raised without any hormones or antibiotics in their feed, and without any DDT residue in the environment. These all-natural dairy products are prime sources of natural lactic acid, a valuable substance which has a beneficial anti-putrefactive and natural detoxifying effect on the digestive and intestinal tracts. This natural lactic acid participates in the life-renewal processes of metabolizing foods and oxygen and casting off waste products.

Note: In civilized countries, a common deficiency of lactic acid means that some body cells and tissues may become clogged with insoluble debris, or "metabolic clinkers," and begin to degenerate. An oxygen-starved cell begins the aging process. It is lactic acid, such as that from all-natural cheese and buttermilk, which helps resist these aging symptoms and promote life-long youth among the Abkhasians.

6. **Most fruits and vegetables are organically grown, freshly picked and eaten raw with all meals.** It is a tradition for Abkhasians to eat fresh fruits (particularly grapes) and fresh vegetables such as tomatoes, cabbage, cucumbers and green onions. They also enjoy baby lima beans, cooked slowly for hours, mashed, and served flavored with a natural sauce made of onions, peppers, garlic and pomegranate juice.

Secret Benefit: Organic, fresh raw fruits and vegetables are prime sources of Vitamin C, which helps alter blood composition and decrease incidence of athersclerosis (almost absent among Abkhasians). Vitamins in these raw foods help prevent unwanted oxidations, and they also help sweep up the undesired wastes, which might otherwise cause cellular death and impede the action of vital enzymes. Vitamins help wash away such wastes and thereby boost energy and help the body renew itself.

7. **Large supplies of garlic are available for daily use either in raw vegetable salads or as snacks.** Garlic has always been prescribed by Eurasian folk physicians; the Abkhasians believe in using it daily. It is known for being a general detoxifying food and for helping to improve the heart's rhythm.

Secret Benefit: Modern scientists report that garlic contains many phytoncides, or ingredients that have natural antibiotic benefits. Garlic is said to help destroy the harmful germs while leaving the necessary intestinal flora intact, as a means of defending the body against germs. This is part of the yin-yang principle of harmonious living. Nature has programmed garlic to nullify harmful bacteria and leave beneficial bacteria untouched.

8. **Honey is used as a natural sweetener; sugar is absent from the Abkhasian diet.** For sweetening herb teas or other beverages, these Eurasian people use natural, organic honey; they abstain from sugar.

Secret Benefit: Honey is a prime source of pollen, the male germ of the plant kingdom. Pollen has some 35% protein of which half is in the form of free amino acids. The powerful benefit here is that the amino acids are immediately assimilated within the body, where they act as building and rebuilding blocks of rejuvenation. The pollen in honey is also a prime source of calcium, phosphorus, magnesium, iron, niacin, pantothenic acid, folic acid, biotin and precious Vitamin B12, as well as vitamins A, C, D and E.

Note: Pollen, as a prime and natural ingredient of organic honey, is the nearest of all foods to a truly complete food. It is reportedly seven times as rich in protein elements (amino acids) as either eggs, cheese or beef. It has natural antibiotic properties, which help destroy harmful bacterial organisms and are said to be a foundation of youth.

9. **Abkhasians enjoy physical activity in their advanced years.** The Abkhasians feel that productive work helps keep them youthful. A local saying is, "Without rest, a man cannot work; without work, the rest does not give you any benefit." It is rare for an Abkhasian to become retired.

Secret Benefit: Enjoyable work helps keep the Abkhasians physically active; they are not overweight because activity helps use up calories and also seems to promote a healthy blood cholesterol level. Abkhasians do what they are capable of doing; when young, they perform strenuous tasks, but when they mature, they accept lighter work. However, no aged are ever seen sitting in chairs for long periods, passive, like "old people." The Abkhasians rest, but they do not retire from life!

10. **For any ailments, folk medicines and herbal healers are used.** The Abkhasians rarely show any signs of illness. They practice an Oriental-inspired and traditional program of folk-herbal medicines and natural healers. If a folk medicine does not promote satisfactory healing, they call in a physician.

Secret Benefit: The Eurasian tradition is to use natural plants for healing. The Abkhasians believe that chemicals or synthetics are inharmonious with the wheel of health, and that they may disrupt any healing processes or create internal disharmony. These artificial healings should be used, tradition declares, only when folk-herbal medicines are not satisfactory.

Other Health Secrets

Abkhasians do not smoke or use tobacco in any form. They drink no coffee. Beverages are natural herbal teas sweetened with natural honey. They listen to the radios that are available, but prefer to go outdoors instead of remaining passively before television sets. Although they use tractors, they prefer horseback; this suggests their love for keeping physically active. Men and women walk with posture that is unusually erect, even into their later years. Most Abkhasians take daily walks of about two miles. They swim in mountain streams; they keep themselves slim.

Characteristic of the Abkhasians is the thickness of their hair which, even if gray, is usually abundant. The very elderly, who may be unable to do heavy plowing or do heavy lifting of loads, keep active by doing weeding, sewing, feeding livestock, working in gardens and going for long horseback rides to do errands and other tasks.

A medical team researching the prime-of-life health of the Abkhasians reported that men were vigorous and fertile, as well as virile, long after the age of 70. Close to two out of every ten Abkhasian women remain fertile until about 55 years of age. Their all-natural living traditions and Eurasian health practices have rewarded them with long, healthy and perpetually-young lifespans.

The Abkhasians may have outdistanced the rest of the world in their successful pursuit of youth at all ages. They have drawn from centuries of traditional folk medicine, Oriental and Eurasian secrets of good living and may well earn the title of being the healthiest people in the world!

IN REVIEW:

1. The forever-young Abkhasians draw secrets from their Oriental and Eurasian predecessors. They are a modern people who use traditional folk healing programs and enjoy youth and vitality up to and into their hundreds.
2. Investigators have discovered ten health secrets that promote the look and feel of youth for these healthy people. Such health secrets are easily used in your own home, from locally available organic foods.
3. The Abkhasians are free from the infirmities of civilized countries because they use organic foods, eat wholesomely and take advantage of herbal medicines and folk healers.
4. You can help boost your health and vitality by following the simple Abkhasian way to long life and perpetual youth.

7

Shiatsu:
Secret Japanese Finger-Pressure
Acupuncture for Natural Relief of
Aches, Pains and Soreness

For several centuries, Japanese folk physicians have been healing common ailments by a *finger-pressure acupuncture* method known as *Shiatsu*. Based upon the Chinese needle-insertion treatment of acupuncture, Shiatsu does not rely upon any penetration or puncture of the skin with needles. Instead, the Japanese folk physicians and modern medical healers have discovered that through careful application of the fingertips, palms and heels of the palms, and through gentle manipulative pressures, a feeling of relief can be experienced for such problems as headache, backache, low back pain, regional aches in the fingers and wrists, arms and legs and other joints and muscles.

Throughout modern-day Japan, there are many healing salons as well as special hospitals where Shiatsu is used to help promote natural healing. Many folk physicians urge their patients to learn the simple finger-pressure acupuncture techniques for home relief, during the absence or inaccessibility of a doctor.

Do-It-Yourself Acupuncture Without Needles

Early Japanese tradesmen who went to China in past centuries learned of the acupuncture method of healing. They were impressed by this traditional method and began investigating the possibilities of improving upon it so that it could be done without the use of needles.

Thus began the discovery of Shiatsu, or finger-pressure acupuncture. It has its roots in the first awareness of acupuncture, as recorded by the Jesuits of the Scientific Mission, who were sent to Peking, China, by King Louis XIV. These Jesuits were impressed with evidences of acupuncture healing and wrote about it extensively in private documents. The Jesuits coined the word "acupuncture" from the Latin *acus,* "needle" and *punctura,* or "puncture." In the year 1671, the European Reverend Father Harvieu prepared a secret document entitled *The Secrets of the Medicine of the Chinese, Consisting in Perfect Knowledge of the Pulse.*

This secret document was copied by Japanese scholars, who delved into the secret of those pressure points throughout the body that held the key to unlocking congestion and promoting healing through natural means. The Japanese were unskilled in the use of needles; many traditional folk physicians held that the body was inviolate and should not be pierced for fear of offending the wrath of the deities. So they sought an all-natural, puncture-free method of acupuncture, using the fingertips and palms of the hands. From this beginning, Shiatsu began to rise as a means of natural self-healing of a wide assortment of common and uncommon body aches and pains.

How Finger-Pressure Acupuncture
Works to Relieve Aches

Oriental physicians who specialize in Shiatsu have discovered that specific meridians (or channels, or ducts) extend internally (believed to be embedded in the muscles) throughout the body in a fixed network. The 365 sites on the skin surface are spots where those meridians emerge on the surface. Shiatsu healers explain to their aching patients that skin points, meridians and viscera are interrelated. All of them naturally harbor the ebb and flow, the harmonious balanced rhythm of yin and yang. If there is a disturbance in bodily health, a symptom is that of an ache. Therefore, Shiatsu physicians explain that the harmonious rhythm must be re-established through gentle pressure on some of these body meridians. This helps balance the yin and yang principles, restore a better blood flow, and ease the ache or pain.

Healing Benefits: Gentle finger pressure is said to either diminish an excess (abundance) or replenish a deficiency, depending upon the specific needs of that body part. Shiatsu works to drain out the stagnated *pneuma,* thereby enabling fresh, health-building *pneuma* to be provided as a substitute. Shiatsu physicians observe that these 365 meridians or pulse points are the "gate-keepers" of their influenced body organs. When there is a symptom of an ache of any sort, the "gate-keeper" must be refreshed through finger pressure, thereby helping to restore health to the connected body part. It is this traditional folk-healing program that has reportedly brought healing relief for many thousands of Orientals and Occidentals who come to modern day Japanese Shiatsu physicians.

How Shiatsu Helps Relieve Headaches and Neck Pains

Hilda S. is subjected to many headaches, particularly a stiffness in the nape of her neck. Much of this is due to the tensions of her work as a bookkeeper and from having to manage a family at home. A well-earned vacation to Japan enabled her to be treated with finger-pressure acupuncture by a Japanese folk physician. He taught her to "do-it-yourself" to relieve headaches at home. Hilda S. performs this simple finger pressure technique whenever she feels an approaching headache or stiffness:

Hands should be comfortably warm; if necessary, soak the hands in comfortably hot water before beginning the treatment. Dry hands and fingers thoroughly. Extend fingers and begin long, firm, even and rhythmic strokes along the sides of the temples. Shiatsu physicians say that the "gate-keepers" of the head are located at these meridians; therefore, use gentle strokes along these meridians to help refresh these "gate-keepers."

Next, stiffen the fingertips and press gently in the slight hollow on the sides of the forehead, around the impressed cavities surrounding the eyes. Gently continue this fingertip pressure while you keep moving your head around and around and backwards. Remember, the Shiatsu rule is to be *gentle* in applying pressure.

Next, work your hands around to the nape of your neck. Gently stroke this area and then use fingertip pressure in the hollow of the nape, beating a very gentle and soothing rhythm. Maintain a uniform type of Shiatsu pressure while you continue the very gentle neck rolling.

Folk healers prescribe about 15 minutes daily of such self-healing to help refresh and replenish the pneuma pockets and enable the yin-yang balance to be restored. This is a standard treatment used by many Shiatsu physicians in modern Japan, and it is known for promoting relief of headaches and neck pains.

Hilda S. did experience relief in Japan when being treated for her recurring headaches. She now follows this same program at home, every single day, and has fewer headaches. She has also experienced merciful relief of those tight "tension pockets" that felt like tied up knots in her head. Simple? Yes. Effective? Most definitely — in accordance with Japanese tradition.

How Shiatsu Helps Relieve Arthritic-Like Leg Pains

To Shiatsu physicians, arthritic-like pains are considered a disturbance of the yin-yang balance. They explain that there are 12 double meridians, each pair placed symmetrically on either side of the body, corresponding to the twelve organs to which traditional Oriental medicine attributes all the bodily functions. Shiatsu physicians explain that energy constantly flows along these meridians or channels; energy goes from a yang organ to a yin organ and vice-versa.

Six of these meridians are yang; they are on the left side of the limbs and correspond to the external yang organs. Six of these meridians are yin; they are on the right side of the limbs and correspond to the internal yin organs.

These 12 meridians need to run in a smooth and harmonious balance. But just as Nature inevitably produces clashes in the environment (storms, hurricanes, earthquakes, etc.), so does Nature frequently cause clashes within the body. Just as Nature often upsets the yin-yang balance of the environment, so does she cause this same yin-yang disturbance among the body's 12 meridians. This creates arthritic-like symptoms — a signal that Shiatsu is required to help restore a disturbed equilibrium between the various factors.

An arthritic-like pain in the lower limbs, for example, is considered by Shiatsu physicians as Nature's signal that harmony is to be restored to the upset meridians or channels. A well-known and time-tested do-it-yourself Shiatsu program for relief of aching leg pains is the following, as derived from a reported situation.

How Michael U. Relieves Leg Aches With Shiatsu: With the guidance of a Shiatsu folk doctor, Michael U. was able to bring about relief from frequently recurring "arthritic-like" leg pains with this traditional needle-free acupuncture program:

1. Fill the tub with comfortably warm water. Use soapy hands as a lubricant. Prop the ball of your left foot against one end of the tub. Now lean forward. Circle your ankle with both hands. Gently press your thumbs on your shinbones. Slowly stroke upward toward your knee. Gradually increase the gentle Shiatsu pressures and strokes, up and down from your ankles to your knee. Continue this same thumb pressure and palm massage from your ankles, up along your calf muscles, then to your knee, for about five minutes.

2. Now, as you sit on the rim of the tub, place both feet on the bottom of the tub but keep your knees bent. Use the bone portions of your thumbs to gently knead beneath your kneecap. At the same time, your fingertips keep up a circular motion around your knee joint. Press deeply, but without any discomfort. (Shiatsu physicians strictly prohibit any self-inflicted discomfort during such treatments. The emphasis is on gentleness and comfortable pressure.) Increase these motions and start the pressure-massage strokes around your thighs. Slowly begin to knead your underthigh muslces. Use steady rotary movements as your thumb bones and fingertips continue this pressure. Continue up to ten minutes.

3. Fingertip press the backs of your upper thighs (gluteal muscles) and move your bone structure back and forth over the fatty and muscular layers of tissues. Slowly move your pelvis in a rotary rhythm as a means of helping to liberate congestion spots and further re-establish the imbalanced energy flow. Continue up to five minutes.

4. Lean back against the sloping end of your tub. Try to place your soles against the other sloping end and push yourself. Grip the tub sides with your hands. Push. Shiatsu folk physicians feel that as you push, you should knead your back muscles by moving your skeletal structure (rib cage and shoulder blades) up and down over them as they are flat against the rear of the tub. This is said to help promote rhythmic harmony and restore a flow of energy throughout the congested limbs, thereby promoting relief and well-being. Continue up to five minutes.

In Conclusion: Shiatsu folk physicians instructed Michael U. to finish by soaking in a warm tub for just five minutes, and to follow this with a comfortably cool, needle-spray shower to rinse off. He was then instructed to rub himself dry with a Turkish towel.

Michael U. has found that this Shiatsu folk treatment has helped to liberate congested pockets in his legs and ease his arthritic-like pains. Folk physicians explain that Shiatsu finger pressure, as used by Michael U., works to promote a toning of the body system as well as a form of natural sedation. The finger pressure calms the corresponding organ by dissipating the excessive energy that led to its disturbance. Finger pressure helps reinforce the benefit of a tonification or sedation point, relieving the symptoms caused by congestion. For hundreds of years, Shiatsu has reportedly helped bring all-natural relief for such arthritic-like disturbances in the legs.

Simple Shiatsu Programs to Relieve Backache

Shiatsu physicians explain that a special yin meridian begins at the sole of the foot and extends up to the collarbone. If there is an excessive yang influence, a disturbance may lead to a symptom such as backache. Shiatsu finger-pressure healing works to either reduce a visceral plethora or supplement a deficiency, depending upon the extremes of the imbalance.

Many Shiatsu physicians have a simple program to help relieve aches of the back.

How Irma V. Enjoys Relief of Backache
With Simple Shiatsu

When Irma V. and her husband attended a locally held business exposition from the Orient, she experienced such backache distress that she could hardly walk erect. A Japanese importer-friend noted her problem, asked about the symptoms, and then suggested that she avail herself of a traditional Shiatsu treatment by a Japanese physician who accompanied the Oriental group.

Here is the program that the Shiatsu folk physician followed to help Irma V. enjoy backache relief:

1. Have the person lie face down. The other person (either a Shiatsu folk physician or an aid who has been taught how to duplicate these natural finger pressures) then begins a series of light peck-peck-peck thumb and fingertip motions along the "indented" spinal column. Action is directed on the border of the spinal column, which tradition holds to be the location of the meridians. Begin at the neck and keep going downward. Continue up to 60 seconds.

2. Place both hands on either side of the base of the spine; the fingers should be flat. Now *gently* press fingertips and heel-of-the-hand portions so as to create a firm manipulation. Move upward over extruding muscles alongside the backbone. Continue going upward and press firmly as you reach the shoulders. Use gentle pressures on the nape of the neck, then pause. Slowly continue downward. Repeat up to five times in either direction.

3. Use fingertip kneading. Begin at the neck vertebrae. Press fingertips firmly against the skin. Now move the muscles in small circles. *Hint:* Modern Shiatsu folk physicians note that the yin-yang principle is more effectively balanced in restoration if the right hand moves clockwise, while the left hand moves counter-clockwise. After five such circles, fingers should move down slowly until the entire back is treated. This is said to free the congested meridians and promote more soothing relief from tensions and back distress.

4. The final stage of the Shiatsu program calls for using

gentle hand pressure up and down the body's length of the spine — but not on the spine. Begin with stronger (but comfortable) pressures and gradually ease up until the entire back is covered.

Finishing Techniques. The Shiatsu physician then suggested that Irma V. go to bed. He also had a modern tip for her (illustrative of the increasing modernization of ancient folk medicine to keep in tune with current knowledge). He noted that she would experience a greater degree of back comfort after the Shiatsu folk healing if she would use a plywood bed board.

Benefit: The physician said that a half-inch plywood panel inserted between the mattress and springs would offer the lumbar muscles a desired amount of resilience and support. This would further help in balancing the yin-yang rhythm, which would promote effective healing. Again we can see that a skillful blending of the ancient Orient and modern civilization can bring about a desired effect.

Irma V.'s husband is able to help relieve her backaches with these programs. Reportedly, the durations of Irma's backaches have been shortened and they are less frequent. Shiatsu has helped replace the rhythm of the yin-yang and, in accordance with traditional Oriental medicine, once that all-important balance has been restored, recovery of normal health may be anticipated.

How to Use Shiatsu to Limber Up Aching Wrists and Arms

Shiatsu physicians explain that a special yang meridian begins at the tip of the forefinger and extends right up to the shoulder and collarbone, and even up to the nostril. If there is an excessive yin influence, then a disturbance may manifest itself in the form of aching wrists and arms. The benefit of Shiatsu finger pressure is to help enable the circulation to act more harmoniously and to "unlock" any congestion. Shiatsu physicians reportedly are able to bring about relief of aching wrists and arms with such simple all-natural and traditional finger-pressure treatments.

How Robert O'C. Uses Simple Shiatsu at Home to Ease Symptoms of Wrist and Arm Stiffness

His work as a blueprint draftsman means that Robert O'C. is often hunched over a drawing table, clutching a variety of writing tools. Tension adds to the pressure. He frequently feels stiffness in his wrists and arms, but scoffs at his co-worker's suggestion that it is arthritis. Instead, he feels it is due to an internal congestion because of his working posture and clutching of writing tools. Robert O'C. once made a business trip to Japan where he was effectively treated for this so-called arthritic-like stiffness by a Shiatsu physician; hence, his reliance upon this all-natural program of healing relief.

The Shiatsu physician taught Robert O'C. to perform these five simple motions to relieve the aching of his wrists and arms:

1. Begin by letting the hands dangle loosely from the wrists. Keep forearms at right angles to your body. Shake your hands vigorously (keep them loose!) up and down up to 60 seconds. Imagine that your hands are wet and you want to shake off all the droplets of water.

2. Sit at a table. Place elbows on the table. Move your forearms down so that your fingers are spread fanwise on the table. With your fingers flat and fanwise and your wrists on the table, raise up your fingers as high as is comfortable. Press down with your fingertips. Make a tight fist with each hand. Relax. Begin again. Repeat up to 12 times.

3. Lift hands from the table. Roll your wrists in an outward motion. Now roll your wrists in an inward motion. Flatten your fingers on the table once at a time. Start with your smaller fingers. The rhythm is similar to playing a piano. Continue up to two minutes.

4. With the thumb and forefinger of the opposite hand, seize the last joint of each finger. Do *not* pull suddenly! Hold comfortably tight and *slowly pull.* Keep doing it until you feel your knuckles are about to crack. Now reverse and push, gripping each part of your finger with your thumb and forefinger. Squeeze gently. Repeat for each finger. Then reverse hands and use the same Shiatsu pressure on the other hand. (*Note:* Modern Shiatsu physicians report that this finger pressure acupuncture is beneficial since it helps improve the flex-

ibility of the tendons — those fibers that work with the muscles in promoting finger flexibility.)

5. A modernized "in office" type of Shiatsu is also prescribed by Japanese folk physicians. Just carry an ordinary rubber ball with you. If possible, have two rubber balls. Whenever you have some spare time, grasp a ball in each hand. Squeeze up to the count of 5, relax for the count of 5, then squeeze again. About a dozen squeezes at different intervals throughout the day should do much to help you loosen up hand and wrist tightness and ease the pains that are often termed "arthritic-like," yet considered imbalanced yin-yang meridians by Shiatsu physicians.

Further Techniques. Modern Japanese folk physicians urge the use of contrasting baths — hot and cold — as a means of boosting sluggish circulation in the hands. They also suggest regular clenching-unclenching of the fists as a means of helping to free congestion along the meridians. Robert O'C. has found these time-tested folk healing programs to be so effective that he is able to work with flexible limbs and welcome comfort.

The Secret Healing Power of Shiatsu

The Shiatsu folk physicians taught that the 12 meridians symbolized 12 rivers that flowed into four seas: the seas of nourishment, blood, energy and bone marrow. A displacement meant that the rivers could not flow freely into the four seas of the body and that this could lead to a disturbance and ill health. Shiatsu finger-pressure acupuncture promotes healing by re-directing the flow of rivers into their proper channels. In modern parlance, it is often said that an imbalanced flow is comparable to internal pollution. Cleanse the pollution and internal health may be achieved.

Japanese Shiatsu healing sought to restore health by proper redistribution of life energy. Folk healers have recognized that some of the meridian's energy could be diverted so that one meridian would have an excess and another would have a deficiency. In such a circumstance, illness could occur. This is based upon the basic foundation of Oriental health, namely, the delicate yin-yang balance.

As an ancient Japanese work on this secret healing has declared, "The energy of the heavens circulates in the heavens in accordance with its own laws, and a man's energy circulates in his body in accordance with the same laws as those of Nature. If that circulation is disturbed, he falls ill." The work then offered the various finger pressure acupuncture techniques such as outlined in this chapter to help restore healthful energy and a balanced feeling of well-being.

Shiatsu is a many-centuries old method of finger-pressure acupuncture. It reportedly acts to restore the balance within the body and ease the arthritic-like pains which are symptoms of the internal disorder. Many have found healing relief from such pains and we may well take note of the importance of the Yin-Yang balance. Shiatsu: another ancient discovery that is finding its way into our modern western science of natural healing.

SUMMARY:

1. Shiatsu is a Japanese form of needle-free, finger-pressure acupuncture, which reportedly provides natural relief of aches and pains of the body. It helps promote relief for aching arms and legs and other body joints.
2. Do-it-yourself acupuncture without needles reportedly healed Hilda S. of the symptoms of her recurring headaches.
3. Shiatsu performed at home helped relieve Michael U.'s arthritic-like leg pains.
4. Irma V.'s husband performs just 3 Shiatsu pressures on her back and is able to help relax and reduce her backache pains.
5. Simple ten-minute Shiatsu finger-pressure movements help Robert O'C. relieve symptoms of wrist-arm-finger stiffness.
6. Shiatsu is a many-centuries-old, traditional folk-healing program that is becoming a needle-free form of acupuncture and is being widely used by naturalists throughout the world. It's traditional Oriental healing. It's natural!

8

Secret Oriental Water Healers for Naturally Rejuvenated Health

For many centuries, Oriental folk physicians have been prescribing water methods for healing and rejuvenation. They
have recognized the natural healing benefits of ocean water
and reported its rejuvenative effects upon patients who had
previously displayed symptoms of premature aging. In the ancient Orient, water was considered one of the sacred healing
elements, as part of a mystical pentagram which included wood,
fire, earth and metal (or minerals) as the other divine principles.
Water was an important link between the components of the
elements, and Oriental folk physicians would often prescribe
ocean water as a secret method of rejuvenation and better
health.

Throughout the South Pacific, right up to our modern times,
these Oriental water-healing secrets are being used as a means
of healthful rejuvenation. It is known that there are some 60
quadrillion tons of dissolved minerals in the oceans of the world,
and these minerals hold one of the keys to better health. The
Orientals have long recognized these "secrets" and prescribed
water healers to those who wanted to recover from the infirmities
of premature aging.

In the many sacred and forbidden Oriental writings, there
are many folk programs that use ocean waters for natural healing,
and many of these secret Oriental "water healers" have been
handed down from generation to generation. The Oriental folk

physicians were very wise in making this discovery, which is now being corroborated by our modern scientists.

Simple Ocean Bathing Helps Promote Youthful Skin

Simple ocean bathing has always been considered a valuable way to help keep a youthful skin texture. The secret here is that the mineral content in sea water contains up to 85% sodium chloride. This helps to regulate the distribution of liquids in body tissues. In particular, sodium chloride attracts *moisture* to the skin, and this is the key to maintaining a youthful texture. A brief soaking or swimming in salty ocean water will do much to help create a magnetic response to skin tissues, which then attracts youth-building moisture. Orientals are known for having smooth, moist skin even in old age, and this may be due to their regular ocean bathing.

Ocean Bathing Puts Body Into Your Hair

Minerals as well as ocean protein are beneficial to the hair shafts of your scalp. A blending of trace minerals with protein helps to give body to the hair.

For hair and scalp conditioning, Oriental folk physicians prescribe a brief swim in the ocean. The hair should *not* be dried in the full sunlight since this may cause breakage. Instead, they suggest drying in the shade. This permits nutrients to become absorbed into the scalp, without excessive drying. Afterwards, they prescribe showering under fresh water to rinse the sticky, salty feeling from the hair. Many modern folk physicians prescribe this simple program to help build better hair health. The enviable, full-bodied hair of the native Orientals who use ocean bathing as a regular traditional healer may well attest to the wisdom of this program.

How Orientals Help Ease Arthritis With Ocean Bathing

Traditionally, Orientals have believed that arthritis is a disorder of the yin-yang principles — a symptom of an internal derangement. Modern Oriental folk physicians will rarely prescribe a dry or warm climate; they realize that the body is deficient in ingredients other than warmth. Instead, they believe that *replacing* the "missing ingredient" will help restore the yin-yang principle and ease arthritic distress. This is where ocean bathing comes in as an Oriental folk treatment.

Iodine Replacement is a Key to Healing. The natural iodine in the ocean water may well be the key to relief of arthritic pain. We know that iodine regulates the acid-alkali balance in the blood and tissues, that it helps to repair and regenerate worn out tissues, that it helps to nourish the skeletal structure, and that it enters into the glandular cells to promote a healthful hormonal balance. In particular, iodine enters into the thyroid gland's secretion. The hormone uses this iodine to nullify germs in the bloodstream and to create a self-cleansing of internal toxemia. Traditional and modern folk physicians of the Orient have said that iodine is needed to create a natural detoxification of such infectious bacteria and thereby bring relief of arthritic symptoms. Many arthritics show a severe deficiency in this iodine mineral. Replacement of iodine through eating ocean plants, as well as through ocean bathing, can do much to correct this imbalance, according to Oriental physicians.

How Margaret McK. Helped Soothe Arthritic Pain With Ocean Bathing at Home

A vacation in the very warm climate of an Australasian island made Margaret McK. feel better, but her arthritic pain was only slightly abated. She had hoped that the soothing warm sunshine and the warming breezes of the Pacific would bring her relief. Like others, she discovered that climate was only a temporary palliative. During a few chilly days, her aching joints painfully manifested themselves and she experienced a knife-like pain when trying to extend her arm to reach for an object on the top shelf of her closet. Twisted over, she managed to make it down to the hotel's dining room. Here, she talked to an Oriental who told her that sea water could be beneficial, that it was a traditional folk healer to restore the internal imbalance.

A Simple Program for Arthritis Relief: Ordinary sea salt is available at almost all health food stores and herbal pharmacies.

Begin by pouring one cup of sea salt into a tub of very hot water. After the sea salt has melted, wait until the tub is comfortably warm. Now, just let yourself relax as your body pores open and the ocean's treasure of minerals from the sea salt begin to seep through the open pores of your skin. Soak yourself for 30 minutes, or longer. Do it nightly. Then, rinse off in a tepid shower, blot yourself dry (don't rub, as this may cause excess stimulation), and then drift off to sleep.

Benefits: Oriental folk physicians of today maintain that the minerals in the sea water, especially iodine, can be absorbed through the skin pores and help correct an internal imbalance. This bath at home, using sea salt, is said to provide comparable benefits to swimming in the ocean.

Results: Margaret McK. reportedly experienced relaxation and relief of her arthritic spasms. Her joints had more flexibility. Her pains subsided. Even in colder weather, she found that she could bear climatic changes with reduced symptoms, when she took this ocean-bathing folk treatment at home.

How Orientals Use a Seaweed Bath to Promote the Look and Feel of Youth

For centuries, aging Oriental potentates would go to secret shrines and hidden sites to undergo rejuvenation under the guidance of mystical and magical folk physicians. The secret of such reported rejuvenation has been mentioned in many of the different Oriental scrolls and writings. It called for taking a "seaweed bath" as a means of restoring internal harmony, thereby permitting a form of self-rejuvenation.

In our modern times, a seaweed bath is often prescribed as a means of regeneration and helping to bring about the look and feel of glowing youth.

Alfred DeN. Feels "Young All Over" With Twice-Weekly Seaweed Baths

Overwork, general neglect of the natural laws of healthful living and an improper diet had all taken their toll on the health of Alfred DeN., an architectural engineer. As a consequence, he experienced cold hands and feet, his skin had an aging pallor, and unsightly wrinkles marred his once-youthful appearance. In particular, he felt distress in the region of his kidneys and liver. Alfred DeN. walked with a stooped gait, was tired by mid-afternoon and had little energy or vitality. When his profession began to suffer because of his inability to work or travel, Alfred decided to go to a health resort. This particular resort prescribed all-natural Oriental methods of healing. Alfred was given daily seaweed baths.

Benefits of Seaweed Baths: Ordinary seaweed is available at health stores and herbal pharmacies (or, you might contact any supplier of fishing supplies and ask if they have seaweed available). Also, many folks will gather up seaweed during a trip to the seashore, pack it in moist towels and bring it home for use in the tub.

Since seaweed derives its nourishment from the ocean, it is a prime source of the sea's nutritional elements. One of the benefits of seaweed is that it provides a certain amount of friction. Rub it against yourself as a "massage glove" when taking a seaweed bath.

When a bunch of seaweed is soaked in a comfortably hot tub, the rich ocean treasure of salt, minerals, vitamins and other substances are released into the water. This makes the tub a veritable treasure of healing ingredients.

Secret Rejuvenation Power: When you soak yourself in a comfortably hot seaweed bath, you undergo increased perspiration. This helps to drain off toxic substances. This is known as "therapeutic sweating," which offers a self-cleansing of internal toxemia and promotes youthful cleansing. This is believed to increase cellular metabolism in many body tissues and cells; as such, it is helpful in restoring the youthful cleanliness of the bloodstream, kidneys, liver and related organs. Such a restoration of harmony is also soothing in problems of arthritis and similar joint-pain conditions.

How Orientals Enjoy Rejuvenation With This Secret

When Alfred DeN. soaked in the tub, he derived the same rejuvenation benefit enjoyed as a sacred secret by the Orientals, namely, *wet heat* helped clean the blood of impurities.

The hotter the skin surface, the greater the rejuvenated activity of the sweat glands in the excretion of urea, uric acid, cholesterol, antibodies, narcotics, and the constituents of bile and urine, which the glands cast off in greater quantities in *wet heat* than when the skin surface is allowed to evaporate in *dry heat.*

How a "Wet Heat" Seaweed Bath Promotes the Feeling of Youth

A 30-minute soak offers this reported benefit. It alerts the sweat glands to create rhythmic cleansing. This helps regulate cholesterol imbalance and also balances the blood fats (often believed to lead to age-causing hardening of the blood vessels). The bath further stimulates sluggish glands to help increase the body's oxygen content (relieving a predisposition to cardiovascular distress) and decrease the carbon dioxide content of the venous blood.

Wet heat stimulation helps remove sugar and acid accumulations, which are problems of diabetes. It also helps relieve problems of acidosis and uric acid.

Many past and present Orientals who discovered this secret rejuvenation program take regular seaweed baths right at home. In the situation of Alfred DeN., he took such a bath at a special salon, and after five folk treatments, he felt remarkably well and was able to bounce back with youthful vitality.

How Orientals Make a Seaweed Bath: Obtain bunches of seaweed from a herbal pharmacy or fishery supplies store. Dump a handful of seaweed or more into very hot water. When the water is comfortable, immerse yourself and remain in it from 30 to 45 minutes. Afterwards, rinse off beneath a tepid shower. You may keep on perspiring afterward, so wrap yourself in a comfortable towel and lie down for a well-deserved rest.

Special Hint: Modern Oriental health salons add a teaspoonful of pine needle extract (available at most herbal pharmacies) to promote a sweet, natural essence. This also helps to promote youthful relaxation and reportedly washes away the feeling of fatigued, aching muscles.

Herbal Bubble Bath: From your herbal pharmacy, obtain any herbal bubble bath powder and mix it with the seaweed. The benefit here is that the bubbles are more than just a luxury — they create an exhilarating, insulating action. The heat of the seaweed-water does not escape into the atmosphere. Instead, the mineral-rich vapors are "sealed" into the body. Thus, metabolism becomes stimulated and oxygen intake is increased. If the bubbly foam is thus maintained, remain in the tub up to an hour. This enables your skin to get the full rejuvenation treatment — *in* and *on* the skin — for healthful, natural results.

To finish, when the water has cooled, rinse yourself quickly under a tepid shower and towel yourself dry.

Overall Benefit: After the treatment, your body will have disposed of stored-up poisons, replaced them with youth-building minerals and alerted your sluggish stimulation so that your glandular network and body processes can work at youthful efficiency. The ancient Orientals considered this to be a sacred secret of rejuvenation. Today, modern folks are discovering that a seaweed bath with herbal bath powders can do much to bring about yin-yang harmony and promote a welcome feeling of youthful health.

Mediterranean Secret of Youthful Skin

Cleopatra, the symbol of ancient beauty, was said to have come across a secret of maintaining youthfulness based upon a mixture of Oriental and Mediterranean folk healing. Her secret was to use any type of fish oil as a skin ointment. After a thorough "oiling" of her skin, Cleopatra would soak herself in a tub of sea water. It is reported in many archives that this secret helped erase any skin blemishes that might otherwise have resulted from the harsh and volatile climate of the Egyptian desert.

Benefits: Fish oils contain ingredients that closely resemble the oils in the skin's sebaceous glands. During youth, these glands secrete an abundance of hormones to help keep the skin looking soft and supple; in later years, however, the glands slow up, and fish oils can be used to replenish human glandular oils. Fish oils also contain disinfectant minerals that help remove impurities such as acne and blackheads. With this, they also provide an astringent action, which helps to tighten up sagging skin tissues.

Although Cleopatra was probably not aware of these scientific facts, she knew that through regular applications of fish oil to her skin she could prevent the wrinkles, dryness and age spots which are often signs of aging. It is said that she rewarded Oriental caravan merchants with precious gems for having given her this secret of healthy, youthful skin.

Ocean Vapors Help Pep Up Metabolism

Dorothy LeC. had breathing difficulties. She was constantly suffering from headaches, felt a tight "tension knot" between her shoulder blades and moved with muscle-stiff difficulty. She had hoped that a vacation in Hawaii would help, but it offered only partial relief. Once, she attended a lecture given by Oriental folk physicians and came away with a secret of rejuvenation that has made her feel as if she were "reborn."

Secret: When swimming in the ocean, or when soaking yourself in a sea-water tub, breathe in very deeply. Oriental healers suggest breathing in and holding the breath to the count of five, then exhaling. The benefit here is that in many mature folks, the lungs become less elastic and the rib cage grows rigid and has less ability to expand fully. Breathing in the mineral-rich vapors of the sea water in the tub will do much to help send a stream of nutrition into the bloodstream, via the oxygen-absorbing system.

As a benefit, this steady breathing of the mineral-rich treasures of ocean vapors will help cast off those waste substances that are often the causes of headaches, backaches and stiff muscles and joints.

Dorothy LeC., swam in the ocean, during which time she devoted up to 15 minutes to deep breathing. This helped to cleanse and stimulate her bloodstream, and to pep up her metabolism. Once her metabolism was invigorated, some of her excess body fat was turned into energy-creating fuel.

So relieved was Dorothy LeC. that she obtained sacks of seaweed from a nearby beach and took regular baths right in her own tub. She added sea salt to create more ocean vapors and breathed deeply, feeling a surge of healthful vitality. This gave her a new lease on life. Her aches became relieved, her energy was boosted and she became more lively and youthful, thanks to this Oriental folk secret, which can be practiced conveniently at home.

Your Equipment: Obtain sacks of dried seaweed from fishery supplies outfits, herbal pharmacies or health stores. Place the seaweed in muslin cloth and make this into a little sack. Let it soak in boiling hot water so that the ingredients can be released in the tub. Wait until water is comfortably cool.

How to Self-Rejuvenate: Soak yourself in the tub. Use the seaweed sack to rub yourself. The benefit here is that you give yourself a friction massage, which helps draw blood to the surface of the skin. This then sloughs off toxic wastes through the pores.

Wastes are drawn up from the kidneys, liver and intestines, and thus are excreted. The secret here is that the warmth enables the capillary blood vessels to expand; this lets the blood circulate more freely throughout the body. Once this is done, the minerals from the seaweed (especially gland-feeding iodine) can penetrate the pores of the skin, disinfect the skin and create a natural feeling of rejuvenation — internally and externally.

To Finish: Rinse off in tepid water and blot yourself dry. Then lie down and rest.

A Seaweed Bath offers "overnight rejuvenation" because the friction massage, together with the infusion of ocean minerals, helps create a tonic effect. This enables the sodium chloride in the water to create body insulation. The minerals are soaked into the body where they work to stimulate metabolism and boost an otherwise sluggish oxygen supply.

This Oriental program also calls for healthful perspiration, which enables the surface cells and tissues to dilate, thus relaxing the blood pressure and easing pressure on the heart. Many Orientals know that this secret healing program is a restorative tonic. It can soothe the nerves and melt stiffness. In brief, it can restore the displaced yin-yang balance and bring harmony to the body. In harmony, there is youth, say the Oriental sages. By using Oriental "water healers," as did the ancient imperial royalists, there is hope for rejuvenation and better health in our modern times.

SPECIAL HIGHLIGHTS:

1. The ocean is a treasure of youth-building vitamins, minerals and proteins.
2. Simple ocean bathing helps rejuvenate the skin and improve the health of the hair.
3. Oriental healers prescribe iodine-rich ocean bathing to relieve arthritic-like distress. Margaret McK. felt soothing relief with ocean bathing right in her own home.
4. A seaweed bath is an ancient Oriental secret for the look and feel of youth. It can be enjoyed right in your own home.
5. Alfred DeN. feels "young all over" with twice-weekly seaweed baths in his own tub.
6. Discover the secret rejuvenation power of a "wet-heat" bath.
7. Cleopatra's secret of "eternal youth" is now shared by modern civilization.
8. Ocean vapors helped boost Dorothy LeC.'s feeling of better health and youth. She creates "ocean vapors" right in her own bathtub by using just one locally available item. A seaweed bath is an Oriental secret of "overnight rejuvenation" that can be enjoyed right in your own home.

9

Korean Ginseng:
Magic Herb for Sexual Power

For over 5,000 years, Oriental Ginseng (known botanically as *Panax schinseng*), has been reverently used by the people of China, Korea, Japan, Southeast Asia, India, Indo-China and Siberian Russia for its vitalizing and restorative powers. Ginseng is a prized magic herb as well as a recognized medicinal asset of the Orientals. Throughout Asia, Ginseng was, and still is, considered to be the most valuable of all medicinal herbs. The Orientals call it the "Magic Rejuvenation Herb for Perpetual Virility." Its enthusiasts consider it the panacea of all ailments. The sick take it to help recover their health; the astute Orientals take it to give themselves the feeling of perpetual virility. The healthy use Ginseng to build up resistance to common ailments and to make themselves stronger and more youthfully alert in body and mind. Oriental Ginseng may well be the one outstanding secret of youthful health that surpasses all other time-tested secrets.

Why Orientals Believe in the Magic
Rejuvenation Herb

Oriental folk physicians have asserted that a plant is effective against ailments of that organ which shape it resembles. Of all their healing plants and herbs, Ginseng was the only one that was shaped like a man. (The shape of the Ginseng root does resemble the arms, legs, trunk and chest of a man.) To the

114

Orientals, this was Nature's secret way of revealing that the Ginseng herb was a prime source of all the elements that would help rebuild a man's health and his powers of virility.

The Oriental Harvesting Tradition Has a Scientific Basis. What started as an Oriental superstition has become a scientific reality in our modern times. For example, the Orientals believed that the Ginseng herb should be harvested or gathered at the "ghost hours," or at midnight, when the heavens were brightened by a full moon. They utilized all the paraphernalia of the magicians of the era in order to perform Ginseng harvesting in an aura of strange mystery. But today, we see that this superstition does have a scientific basis: *many medicinal herbs, particularly Ginseng, do retain their active ingredients only as long as the dew has not dried on their leaves.* The ancient Oriental physicians were aware of this, and they decreed a special ritual that required the Ginseng root to be dug out only at midnight, in the presence of a full moon. As such, the harvested Ginseng possessed its valuable youth-building properties because the dew was still moist upon the leaves.

So we see that this ancient, magical superstition does have a valid scientific basis. To this day, Orientals prize midnight-harvested Ginseng as possessing the "magic ingredients" to help promote perpetual vitality and virility.

The name *Ginseng* was coined by the Oriental physicians from two words meaning "man plant." The generic name of Ginseng, or *Panax,* is derived from the Greek word "panacea," meaning cure-all. For centuries, the Asians have considered this "man plant" to be a cure for most ailments and infirmities.

Love Potion, Revitalizer, Rejuvenator

During the second millennium B.C., the Oriental ruling dynasty, the Shang family (later called the Yin dynasty), wrote about the magic powers of the Ginseng herb. They wrote their findings on bones which were excavated during the 20th Century in the northern region of what is currently known as the province of Honan. The Shang-Yin dynasty folk physicians recorded the secrets of the Ginseng root and told of how it could increase one's lovemaking power, while helping to promote a feeling of revitalization as well as rejuvenation.

Between the 10th and 6th Centuries B.C., various folk physicians were mentioned in a great collection of Oriental secrets called *Shih Ching,* or the *Book of Songs.* Writing in the form of lyrics, folk physicians listed various ailments that could be healed with the use of the magic Ginseng herb. They told of the various people who were remarkably revitalized by the magic power of this all-natural herb.

The noted Huang-ti Nei-ching extolled the magic youth powers of Ginseng in his *Yellow Emperor's Classic of Internal Medicine.* He, too, used the Oriental lyric writing style in explaining how this simple yet "magic" herb could produce youthful healing in men and women of all ages.

About 2,500 years ago, Oriental folk physicians recorded many case histories of the youth-building benefits of Ginseng in many documents. This herb is revered as a "magic power" in the *History of the Late Han Dynasty* (Hou Han Shu), as well as in the medical work, *Encyclopedia of the Emperor Tai Tsung (T'aip'ing Yii Lan),* and also in the *Imperial Encyclopedia (Ku-chin T'u-shu Chi-ch'eng)* published in 1726 A.D. These documents summarized the full range of scientific and medical knowledge, which is so surprisingly current that modern Oriental physicians consider them to be immortal for their health secrets. These books, and many others, consider Ginseng to be the most effective herb in helping to create a feeling of youthful health.

Hailed as an Aphrodisiac. Li Shih-chen, the highly respected Oriental physician and pharmacologist who lived towards the end of the 16th century, hailed Ginseng root as an aphrodisiac and love philter and recommended it highly for a variety of ailments in his noted *Pharmacopoeia* (Pen-ts'ao Kang-mu).

Health Benefits of Ginseng: The noted Li Shih-chen, regarded as the Great Healer, wrote that Ginseng could "rejuvenate the five senses, restore the well-being of the soul, soothe fears, help cast out the demons, refresh the eyes, strengthen the heart, rebuild understanding and knowledge, remake the body, restore the stamina of a bridal couple and promote the joy of productive livelihood." From this poetic style, we can deduce that he referred to Ginseng as containing the magical properties that would help heal imfirmities, promote a feeling of reactivated health and emotional and mental vigor, and that it would promote virility in males and females. Dr. Li Shih-chen listed many case histories attesting to the "magic youth" power of Ginseng.

The Appearance of the "Man Plant": The Ginseng root is, as was mentioned before, similar to the human body. The two tips of the root resemble legs; its two upper continuations resemble arms. It is basically a wild plant that requires a moist, darkened, humus-filled earth in order to thrive. Above ground, the Ginseng plant has a few leaves and a strange green-white blossom. While this, too, may be used as a potion, it is the root that has always been highly prized for its youth-building powers.

More About the Herb of Eternal Life

Nearly all Oriental physicians and scholars who have investigated the magic powers of Ginseng have reported that its secret is not solely to help create a surge of virility. Ginseng is reportedly able to revive, restore and reactivate the entire body and thereby help to invigorate the organism as a whole. A regenerated body is able to send forth an ample supply of hormones to the reproductive glands, thereby creating an aphrodisiac type of benefit. The Orientals of the past and the present were wise to realize that a healthy body can serve its owner with perpetual virility. Ginseng was said to help boost body health and thereby enable it to function with virile health.

When Marco Polo voyaged through the Orient in approximately 1275 A.D., he reported that Ginseng was used by many who sought to heal their infirmities and enjoy a restoration of youthful health.

A Modern Discovery. Sir Edwin Arnold, the famous Orientalist scholar, author of *The Light of Asia,* traveled throughout the regions where Ginseng was used and discovered it to be most beneficial for its restoration of youth and vigor. He states:

"According to the Chinese, Asiatic Ginseng is the best and most potent of all Cordials, Stimulants, Tonics, Stomachics (digestive tonics), Cardiacs, Febrifuges (fever reducers) and, above all, will best renovate and reinvigorate failing forces.

"It fills the heart with hilarity, while its occasional use will, it is said, add a decade to human life. Have all these millions of Orientals, all these many generations of men, who boiled Ginseng in silver kettles and praised heaven for its many benefits, been totally decieved? Was the world ever quite mistaken when half of it believed in something never puffed, never advertised and not yet fallen to the fate of a trust, a Combine or Corner?"

American Report. The United States Consul at Seoul, Korea, in its U. S. Consular Report No. 65, officially reports that "From personal experience and observation I am assured that Korean Ginseng is active, strongly-heated medicine. Western people appear to regard the virtues of Ginseng claimed by the Orientals rather contemptuously — as imaginary and based on superstition. The evidence is that the mystic value attached itself to Ginseng after its virtues have been practically ascertained."

More Youth Restorative Benefits of Ginseng

The medical reporter, Paul M. Kourennoff, in his exhaustive work, *Russian Folk Medicine,* says the following about the youth restorative benefits of Ginseng:

"It was taken in hemiopathic (almost full strength) doses, either in the form of an alcoholic infusion, or powder (usually in combination with some other medicinal herbs), and the prolonged use was said to cause gray hair to turn black, new teeth to grow, and all wrinkles to disappear. Some old men of 89 and 90 were said to become vigorous enough to take young wives and sire children, but all these claims have never been medically confirmed.

"What was confirmed by all European doctors practicing in the Orient was that the use of Ginsing medications had an extraordinary effect upon the metabolism of all takers, and dramatically improved the general tonus of their systems.

"It was not unusual for very old men in China to marry and have children, and to boast openly of their sex prowess. All such ancient Casanovas attributed this to the use of Ginseng."

Soviet Union Praises Ginseng Powers. In the later 1930's, scientists of the Institute of Experimental Medicine in the

U.S.S.R. were sent to the Orient to see, first hand, if Ginseng could produce the remarkable rejuvenation benefits as reported. Their findings are summarized in the *Cyclopedia Dictionary of Medical Botany,* by C. S. Ogolevec:

"During the Korean War, millions of dollars' worth of Korean Ginseng were sent to the U.S.S.R. when the northern armies overran Korea. The Soviet scientists investigated the properties of this Ginseng and found that many of the things the Orientals were saying about Ginsing were true. They gave its structure as $C_{32}H_{36}O_{49}H_{48}O_3$ stating among other properties that it strengthens the heart and the nervous system and increases the hormones, etc. It contains Panaxin, Panaquilom, Schingenin, etc."

Soviet scientists have already cultivated fields in the region of South Siberia, and are reportedly growing full "plantations" of Ginseng which they hope may hold the secret of perpetual virility.

Modern Secret of Ginseng Power: It has been reported by scientists that Ginseng emits a *mitogenetic* ray which is considered an all-natural, ultra-violet radiation. Nature has put within the Ginseng herb a process of cellular proliferation via this mitogenetic emission. It is said that this all-natural cellular rejuvenation process stimulates the body's own sluggish processes and thereby promotes the youth-building benefit of cellular renewal — the key to healing and regeneration. This modern scientific discovery corroborates the ancient Oriental awareness of the youth-building powers of Ginseng.

Sexual Vigor Restored by Ginseng. Paul M. Kourennoff, in his reputable *Oriental Health Secrets,* tells of asking a San Francisco Oriental physician for a good Chinese-Tibetan folk remedy for the treatment of sexual impotence. Dr. S. N. Chernych reportedly said:

"Ginseng! Oriental healers are successfully curing patients of sexual impotence by the use of Ginseng, and sexual impotence is one of the most difficult disorders. I can state from personal experience, that the Oriental physicians have cured several men whom I and several other doctors tried to help."

Reported Case Histories. Paul M. Kourennoff, then relates:

"The author can verify this from his own personal observations in the city of Harbin, Manchuria, during the years 1920-

1923. Harbin was crowded with civilian refugees and interned units of the Russian National (White) Army. Most of these ex-soldiers had served in the First World War, and later in the Civil War (referring to the Russian Revolution). Nerve-shattered and ill, many of these veterans were suddenly stricken with sexual impotence.

From Impotence to Instant Virility. "They stormed the offices of regular doctors of medicine and, receiving no help, finally turned to the Chinese healers. It is reported that all of them were cured by the Chinese practitioners, chiefly with the aid of ginseng, occasionally supplemented by, or combined with, other substances. Three of six persons known to the author were completely cured (of impotence) by the use of ginseng alone.

Magic Power of Sexual Vigor. "When all else has failed to restore sexual vigor, Ginseng can be counted on, if there is any hope at all. There is nothing mysterious or supernatural about its curative properties. No one need fear its use if directions are followed carefully. We should think no more of taking a dose of Ginseng for sexual impotence than taking a dose of castor oil for constipation, for Ginseng is as much a vegetable as the castor bean."

A Doctor Tells of the Magic
Healing Power of Ginseng

One of the earliest Western studies given to Ginseng was made by a reputable physician, A. R. Harding, M.D., who possessed an unbiased attitude toward traditional Oriental healing secrets. He made a cautious study of Ginseng and began prescribing the Oriental plant to his patients. He was so enthused over its results that he began growing Ginseng, which he then harvested according to traditional Oriental custom and gave to his ailing patients. In Dr. Harding's work, *Ginseng and Other Medicinal Plants,* he tells of the magic healing power of this Oriental herb:

"For several years I have been experimenting with Ginseng as a medical agent and of late I have prescribed, or rather added it to, the treatment of some cases of rheumatism.

"I remember one instance in particular of a middle-aged man who had gone the rounds of the neighborhood doctors and failed to find relief; then he employed me. After treating him for several weeks and failing to entirely relieve him, more especially the distress in bowels and back, I concluded to add Ginseng to his treatment. After using the medicine, he returned, saying the last bottle had served him so well that he wanted it filled with the same medicine as before.

"I attribute the curative powers of Ginseng in rheumatism to the stimulating to healthy action of the gastric-juices, causing a healthy flow of the digestive fluids of the stomach, thereby neutralizing the extra secretion of acid that is carried to the nervous membranes of the body and joints, causing the inflammatory condition incident to rheumatism."

How to Take Ginseng

Dr. Harding suggests, "Ginseng combined with the juices of a good ripe pineapple is excellent as a treatment for indigestion. It stimulates the healthy secretion of pepsin, thereby insuring good digestion without incurring the habit of taking pepsin or after-dinner pills to relieve the fullness and distress so common to the American people."

Helps Relieve Coughs. Dr. Harding tells of a lady who had severe coughing which could not be relieved by any medicine. He prescribed Ginseng and it healed her. It loosened her cough, says the doctor, and thereby lessened throat pressures and constrictions, which eventually promoted healing.

Ginseng Tea Heals Chronic Cough. Dr. Harding cites another case:

"A neighbor lady had been treated by two different physicians for a year for a chronic cough. I gave her some Ginseng and told her to make a tea of it at meal times and between meals. In two weeks, I saw her and she told me that she was cured and that she never took any medicine that did her so much good, saying that it acted as a mild cathartic and made her feel good. She keeps Ginseng in her house now all the time and takes a dose or two when she does not feel well."

Different Ginseng Varieties for Your Use

While Ginseng is cultivated all over Asia and America, the Korean Ginseng is reputed to be the most effective. Here are the different Ginseng varieties available for your use:

1. Korean Ginseng (Panax Ginseng). This is grown in high and deep mountains. The cultivation requires a full six years of ceaseless attention. Korean Ginseng is sensitive to the various geographic conditions such as clean air, proper humidity, suitable temperature, special quality of soil and abundant water. It does *not* grow if subjected to chemical or artificial fertilizers. It will not grow in the same place again for ten years after the previous cultivation. Korean Ginseng gardens are registered by law as to the width and length of the bed. Government officials are especially appointed to see how the Ginseng is grown, to know how many roots are available at harvest time. Every grower must sell his entire crop to the government when it is six years old.

2. Korean White Ginseng (Baik-Sam, Ginseng Radix Alba). This Ginseng is prepared by the process of washing, trimming of lateral and fibrous root, and drying. It is not a Korean Government monopoly, but under the strict supervision of quality by the Korean Ginseng Association.

3. American Ginseng (Panax quinquefolius). This is a fleshy-rooted herb native to cool and shady hardwood forests from Quebec to Manitoba, south to Northern Florida, Alabama, Louisiana and Arkansas. Wild Ginseng has been harvested for many years and is cultivated commercially for its root, both in its natural range and in the Pacific Northwest. American Ginseng shows variations in characteristics, particularly in the roots. Western types usually have long, thin roots of undesirable qualities. Plants from the northern part of the country, particularly Wisconsin and New York, are the most desirable for export, furnishing roots of good size, weight and shape, and are generally considered the best breeding stock. Cultivated roots are usually heavier and more uniform than wild roots, although they command a lower price in the market.

Note: The best quality root of proper age breaks with a somewhat soft and waxy fracture. Young or undersized roots dry hard and glassy and are less marketable. *Only whole roots are acceptable to the Oriental.*

Where to Buy Ginseng

Inquire at your local health food shop or ask your neighborhood herbal pharmacy. Mail order companies that supply Ginseng are these:

Herb Products Co., Inc.
11012 Magnolia Boulevard
North Hollywood, California 91601

Golden Gate Herb Research
P.O. Box 77212
San Francisco, California 94107

New Pacific Products Co.
4064 Marchena Drive
Los Angeles, California 90065

Superior Trading Co.
867 Washington Street
San Francisco, California 94108

Gae Poong Korea Ginseng
40-15 150th Street
Flushing, New York 11354

Kiehl Pharmacy Inc.
109 Third Avenue
New York, New York 10011

Ye Olde Herbal Shoppe
8 Beekman Street
New York, New York 10038

The Easy Way to Use Ginseng

The different ways to use Ginsing are these:

1. **Chew the root.** The hard and dry root can easily be sliced into pieces if you first steam it for about five to ten minutes. For adults, about five sliced pieces (about 1 teaspoon) daily, or every other day will be sufficient. Many Orientals carry Ginseng and will chew on it throughout the day.

2. **Ginseng Elixir.** Grate the dried root until it is a powder. Mix one-half teaspoon with a cup of boiled water and add a natural herb flavor such as cinnamon. Sip slowly.

3. **Ginseng Tonic.** Mix one-half teaspoon Ginseng powder with fresh fruit juice. Stir vigorously and drink slowly.

4. **Ginseng Blossom Tea.** Many Orientals find themselves feeling more buoyant and youthful with this tea. To make it, use the blossom umbels or the dry leaves. Steep these leaves in water, as you would with ordinary teas. Add a bit of honey for flavor. A Ginseng Blossom Tea is a healthful coffee substitute, and it can build good health and a feeling of youthful vigor.

How Ginseng Helps Promote Perpetual Vitality

The secret of Ginseng is in its ability to increase resistance of the body to unhealthy infection. (This benefit is the basic principle of the yin-yang healing program, in which the imbalance has to be restored so that the *cause* is healed, in order to remove the *symptoms*. Ginseng reportedly helps strengthen this delicate youth-building yin-yang balance.)

Ginseng increases the body's resistance to various etiological (causes) factors that might cause ill health. Ginseng acts as a legendary "Chinese Wall of resistance" to excessive cold, heat, radiation, fatigue, toxic-narcotic chemical pollutants and many biological adversities.

Unique Benefit. The most unique and important benefit of Ginseng is its normalization action, which helps create internal harmony. It is able to bring about an internal *balance* of upheavals to restore the yin-yang balance of health.

In particular, Ginseng reportedly helps heal the nervous system, improves the blood pressure, controls cholesterol metabolism so as to resist arteriosclerosis, assists in sugar metabolism, protects the liver, regulates body weight, and helps create energy to normalize the sexual functions.

Secret Oriental Formulae for Health Rejuvenation With Ginseng

Here are some secrets from the Orient, using Ginseng for specific needs:

Basic Health Rule: When cooking Ginseng (or any herb), your utensils should be either glass or earthenware. Do not use any utensils made of metal. When cutting herbs, use wooden tools; do not use metal knives. Mortars in which Ginseng or other herbs are ground should not be made of metal. For storing, use crockery, but do not use metal utensils; glassware is considered the best.

To improve Digestion: Make Ginseng into a powder and dissolve it in the white of an egg. Take this Oriental formula at least three times a day.

To Improve the Heart: Blend one-half teaspoon of pulverized Ginseng with melted butter, oil or margarine. Dissolve this mixture in wine (or fresh fruit juice) and drink twice daily.

Nightcap: Make a light broth of Ginseng powder and any fresh raw vegetable juice. Drink one cup about an hour before retiring.

To Help Rejuvenate Body Organs: Take a half-teaspoon of minced raw Ginseng, several times throughout the day.

To Boost Sluggish Blood Circulation: Mix Ginseng powder with some honey and cinnamon. Eat with a spoon, several times a day.

For "Night Romance": Orientals believe that virile powers are exhilarated by mixing chopped Ginseng root with dried and diced (organic) orange peel. Sweeten with honey. Swallow before "attending to your loved one," say Oriental herbalists and specialists in natural aphrodisiacs.

To Ease Joint Stiffness: Prepare an infusion of two parts Ginseng and one part alfalfa seeds and sip on an empty stomach.

Youth Restoration Tonic: For those who feel weak, or who are troubled with a decline in sexual functions, Oriental folk healers and specialists in aphrodisiacs suggest this tonic: mix raw ginger powder with honey and powdered Ginseng. Add some fresh fruit juice. Steam very slightly. Add hot water in which natural brown rice has been cooked. Drink as a youth-restoration tonic, throughout the day.

The Secret Ingredients of this Magic Youth Herb

This wonder herb, which has been prized for over 5,000 years, has been carefully studied by modern scientists. It has been found that the magic youth herb contains these seven secrets of rejuvenation:

1. *Resin* is a natural organic substance that promotes a cerebro-circulatory electrolyte reaction. This stimulates sluggish functions.

2. *Saponin* is a hygroscopic glucoside which acts as a source of energy for so-called ailing organs.

3. *Starch* in its natural root form creates a process of natural metabolism-assimilation, to nourish internal-external organs.

4. *Tannin* is a soluble astringent phenolic substance, which promotes internal healing of inflammation and a general soothing of the body parts.

5. *Aromic bitters* are minute but healing ingredients which help in the process of assimilation of nutrients.

6. *Volatile oils* are Ginseng juices, created by Nature, to help create a smooth metabolism and to provide lubrication and flexibility for sluggish tissues and cells.

7. *Panacin* is a mysterious but scientifically identified substance in Ginseng that is known for promoting remarkable healing, cellular rejuvenation, tissue regeneration and a strange reactiviation of so-called sluggish arterio-venous portions of the body. Panacin is considered to be the most beneficial of all the ingredients of Ginseng.

A Modern Understanding of the "Secret" Rejuvenation Power of Ginseng

Science has discovered that Ginseng contains several enzymes which are known for promoting a feeling of rejuvenation as well as a regeneration of the brain cells. In particular, Ginseng is believed to provide two valuable enzymes: (1) *Acetylcholine,* which stimulates a nerve cell to generate a small electric charge, which is transmitted to the next cell and carries messages back and forth from the brain. (2) *Cholinesterase,* which enables the nerve to rest, recuperate and recharge itself. Without this second enzyme, believed to be possessed by Ginseng, the brain nerves and other nerves would soon be exhausted and burned out.

It is believed that Ginseng sends these two valuable all-natural ingredients into the system. They offer speedy, coordinated reflexes, rejuvenate the memory storage facilities and assist in many other functions of a healthy nervous system. These two compounds, acetylcholine and cholinesterase, both work to become intimately involved in the youthful activity of the cerebro-neuron system. This causes a triggering of various emotional and physical responses that manifest themselves in feelings of rejuvenation and perpetual virility.

Super-Plus Benefit: Modern science knows that this enzymatic activity secret of Ginseng helps to rejuvenate and reactivate the *entire organism,* as a whole. Since the entire organism needs to be recharged in order to create a feeling of virility, Ginseng offers this super-plus benefit to help boost strength and health.

This corroborates the ancient writings about Ginseng's secret power; namely, that it is more than just an aphrodisiac for the sex organs. It is, instead, Nature's "youth tonic" for the entire body so that sexual health can be enjoyed by the mind as well as by the body.

Today, the original habitat of Ginseng is considered to be the Korean peninsula, which has the most suitable environmental conditions of Nature. Even in Korea, there are only limited regions that are conducive to such cultivation. Ginseng may be grown in other countries, but the soil and climate of these countries are regarded as inferior to that of Korea. There is no doubt that the natural shape, fragrance and therapeutic efficacy of Ginseng from other countries can hardly equal that of Korean Ginseng. The mild climate, the dry, clear weather, the natural shade, the natural fertilizer, the careful cultivation, all add up to healthy Ginseng — the magic herb for perpetual virility.

HIGHLIGHTS:

1. A herb that was prized for 5,000 years as a secret virility food is widely used in our modern times.
2. Ginseng is a reputed Oriental love potion, revitalizer and rejuvenator.
3. Ginseng possesses ingredients to help lengthen life, invigorate weakness, strengthen the heart and nervous systems and create a natural cellular rejuvenation by its mitogenetic rays.

4. Many impotent men reportedly regain virile powers by taking Ginseng.
5. An American physician reports miraculous healing through the Ginseng herb, which he prescribed for his patients.
6. Ginseng is easy to use in any of the recommended methods. Orientals use Ginseng in a variety of described formulae for healing-rejuvenation and perpetual virility.

10

Oriental Secrets of Youthfully Healthy Skin and Hair

The forever-youthful condition of the skin and hair of the Orientals has always aroused the envy of the Western world. The Orientals have learned that Nature can help promote healing as well as provide a rich treasure of youth-building secrets of the skin and hair. For thousands of years, Oriental folk physicians have created "magic rejuvenation" for their patients by sharing these secrets of all-natural youth restoration. These traditional secrets have been handed down from generation to generation throughout the centuries, and today, the modern Oriental is living proof of the rejuvenation powers in all-natural folk programs. Many of these secrets have been shared with Westerners and are slowly being recognized as the natural way to help promote youthfully healthy skin and hair.

16 Oriental Secrets of Using Salt as a Natural Youth Aid

Madge P. always carried a kit of cosmetics, lotions, powders, pills and appliances whenever she made a trip to the South Pacific. Although she was in her forties, Madge P. looked much older. The various skin and hair lotions and cosmetics did little more than to mask the aging that could not be eased by these chemically based embellishments.

How a Polynesian Airline Hostess
Offered the Oriental Secret of Youth

A Polynesian airline hostess helped Madge P. with her suitcase. When it fell open, the array of bottles and boxes fell out. Together, they gathered it all together. The hostess looked youthful; she had clear skin and shining hair. When Madge P. said that she wished she knew the Oriental secret of youthfulness, the hostess took a small box from her bag. In the box, said the Polynesian hostess, was the "secret" of Oriental youthfulness. It contained salt. She explained that ancient folk physicians looked to the surrounding oceans and seas for a treasure of health secrets. They suggested salt from the oceans as a natural healer and a promoter of youthful skin and hair. The Polynesian hostess then shared a set of sixteen different Oriental secrets from the past and from the present. Madge P. tried most of them and soon she, too, carried salt as her only beauty aid. She discovered that ordinary table salt (or sea salt) can do wonders for the health of the skin and hair. Soon, she looked and felt youthful enough to make other people envy her smooth skin and youthful hair. Here are these 16 secrets:

Secret #1. For an excellent mouth wash, use one teaspoon of salt in a glass of warm water. Salt can also be used as a natural dentifrice to help whiten the teeth, harden the gums and sweeten the breath.

Secret #2. To relieve a sore throat, gargle with a teaspoon of salt in a glass of hot water.

Secret #3. Bathe tired eyes in a warm solution of 1/2 teaspoon of salt to a pint of water.

Secret #4. Relieve puffiness around the eyes by applying pads wrung out of a solution of a pint of hot water and one teaspoon of salt. Lie back and relax while this Oriental secret works its healing wonders.

Secret #5. For glossy, shining hair, try this dry shampoo: mix 1 ounce of powdered orris root (available at most herbal pharmacies) with 1/2 pound of salt. Rub well into the scalp; then brush out briskly.

Secret #6. Stimulate your scalp and get rid of embarrassing flakiness with a pack made of 1 cup of salt and 5 tablespoons of water. Rub this paste into your scalp, let it remain for 5 minutes, then remove by brisk brushing and a shampoo.

Secret #7. To help rejuvenate red, wrinkled hands, soak for five minutes in a basin of warm water to which 3 tablespoons of salt has been added.

Secret #8. Soak tired, aching feet in a warm bath to which a generous handful of salt has been added. If feet are especially sore, soak them alternately in a hot salt brine and comfortably hot water. *Tip:* Massage gently with moistened salt to remove dry skin, rinse in cool water and dry thoroughly. Dust with talcum or foot powder.

Secret #9. For a youthful facial, or to clear up a fading tan, mix equal portions of salt and olive oil. Gently massage face and throat with long upward strokes. Let the mixture remain for five minutes, then remove with a facial cloth. Wash your face with mild soap and water or a skin lotion.

Secret #10. To relieve fatique, relax for ten minutes or more in a tub of warm water into which you have tossed several handfuls of salt.

Secret #11. To help relieve nervous tension and stimulate a sluggish circulation, relax in a warm bath for 5 minutes, then give yourself a vigorous massage with generous applications of dry salt. Rinse off in cool water.

Secret #12. Ancient and modern Orientals (especially the Japanese) are known for taking luxury baths as a means of promoting youthful health. Many modern Japanese make their own luxury bath salts. Here's how: spread table salt or rock salt in a flat tin pan. Moisten with a mixture of alcohol, cologne and a few tablespoons of fruit juice for a pleasing color. Let stand, stirring frequently, until alcohol and perfume evaporate, then pack in an apothecary jar or other attractive container. Use as a healthful bath salt that will make your skin glow with the look and feel of Oriental youth.

Secret #13. For any sprains or bruises, make a warm fomentation: dissolve 2 tablespoons of salt in a cup of warm water; mix with some vinegar. Use this as a wet compress. A rough turkish towel is best. A warm fomentation enables the salt to relieve congestion and promote better healing of unsightly blemishes.

Secret #14. To help relieve unsightly boils or growths, ancient and modern Oriental folk physicians suggest this secret: dissolve 1 tablespoon of Epsom salts and 1 tablespoon of salt in a cup of boiled water. Apply as a comfortably hot compress to the affected region as often as possible. It is said to help create healing and restore youthful skin texture.

Secret #15. Troubled with nasal congestion, such as that from a cold or an allergy? Ancient folk physicians prescribed this all-natural nose-drop formula: dissolve a few grains of fine salt in a tablespoon of warm water. Just five or six drops up each nostril reportedly helps ease congestion of the nasal passages and promote better breathing.

Secret #16. For unpleasant or premature blemishes on the skin (and also for sprains or other discolorations), heat up coarse, dry salt in a skillet. When hot, *carefully* pour the dry salt into a very heavy cloth, or a clean stocking. Then *carefully* apply to the affected region and let it remain there until the salt cools off. Repeat throughout the day.

The Orientals have always looked to the oceans for secrets of youth and health, they have harvested the plants and sea-food for nourishment for centuries. They have also harvested the salt for their secrets of youthful skin and hair. Today, this time-tested ancient folk medicine is helping to reactivate and restore youthful health for modern people, just as it did for the ancients.

How Orientals Use a Simple
Fruit for Natural Rejuvenation

An ordinary fruit, available at almost every corner market, has been used for centuries by youthfully healthy South Sea islanders as a beauty treatment. This simple fruit is the *lemon*. Its tart and natural fruit acid helps restore the natural acid mantle of the skin (known as pH) that is so often washed off by alkaline soaps. Yet the "bloom of youth" upon the skin of the happy, alert and glowing South Sea islanders is living proof of the benefits of using lemons as a beauty secret.

Ten Secrets of Using the
Lemon as a Youth Restorative

For centuries, South Sea folklore has given praise to the benefits of the lemon as a youth restorative. Here are ten secrets from the Pacific islanders on using the lemon for helping to create forever-youthful health, internally and externally:

Secret #1. To help cleanse stained or blemished skin, rub the area with a fresh slice of lemon. Let the juice soak into the skin. Let it remain overnight, if possible.

Secret #2. To add brightness to your hair, use a lemon rinse. Strain fresh lemon juice into cool water and rinse your hair several times. Finish with a rinse in clear water.

Secret #3. Rub dry or scaly skin with the peel of a lemon. The lemon oils help to restore your skin to a youthfully silky softness.

Secret #4. Try to soften rough elbows by rubbing the region with the cut side of a lemon.

Secret #5. For rough, chapped or "dishpan" hands, try rubbing the skin with fresh lemon juice after dishwashing or other chores. It helps restore the natural acid mantle, which is removed in washing.

Secret #6. For a sore throat, mix some lemon juice and honey with boiled water. Either gargle or drink this folk potion.

Secret #7. South Sea islanders are noticeably free of acne and blackheads. An Oriental secret is to rub lemon juice directly onto an affected area and allow it to dry. Mix equal portions of lemon juice and rose water (the islanders usually steep a few rose petals in hot water, but Westerners can obtain rose water at most herbal pharmacies). Apply this lotion morning and night. It is said to help heal blemishes and bring about an improved skin condition.

Secret #8. To help lighten freckles, Polynesians have this folk secret: mix one tablespoon of lemon juice with one tablespoon of rose water. Mix in a small amount of powdered Elder flowers (available at most herbal pharmacies) to make a smooth paste. Apply to blemishes and let remain overnight. It is said to help lighten these unsightly blemishes and give the cheeks a floral bloom!

Secret #9. To soften the area around the nails or cuticles of the hand, rub daily with fresh lemon juice.

Secret #10. To help whiten and strengthen the fingernails, rub regularly with a lemon peel.

To the Oriental, the fruit of the lemon tree is a natural youth restorative. In our modern times, the lemon and its fresh juice has been used to help promote healing and restore the bloom of youth to the skin and hair.

The Oriental Herbal Face-Lift That Smoothes Away Wrinkles

Lena Z. marveled at the exquisite beauty and youthful skin of the Japanese maids who worked in the hotel in which she was vacationing. She wondered of their secrets of smooth, glowing skin and vital energy. She learned a traditional Oriental secret from one maid, who said that it was a blending of the past with the present. Lena Z. was given this Oriental herbal face-lift formula:

Steep a handful of rosemary leaves or seeds (organic rosemary tea is satisfactory) in a cup of boiled water for 15 minutes. Strain. When cool, add 1 teaspoon powdered milk and 1 egg white to the tea. Mix, but do *not* beat. Store in your refrigerator. The next night, apply it and let it remain on the skin and throat overnight. This helps tighten up sagging skin, tightens up pores, and invigorates the cells. The mixture then attracts and holds water, which provides a moisturizing benefit. Since youthful skin depends upon its supply of moisture, this herbal face-lift reportedly helps attract water beneath the skin, and promote a plumping-up of sagging cells. This is the Oriental way to smooth and rejuvenate the skin through a natural face lift.

Lena Z. tried the program and experienced such a youthful restoration that now she uses no other cream or lotion; instead, she relies upon this natural face-lift — the centuries-old youth secret from Japan.

How Orientals Exercise the Skin for Youthful Rejuvenation

For centuries, Oriental folk physicians have prescribed skin exercises to help replenish starved tissues and cells and firm up sagging skin. Today, in almost every modern Oriental health salon, simple facial massages are considered part of the rejuvenation program sought by so many Westerners.

To the Oriental, self-massage or self-exercising of the skin is a traditional and natural way to youthful rejuvenation. The skillful Oriental has taken this folk secret and applied it to our modern times. You may use a comfortably stiff complexion brush (sold at all variety stores, many supermarkets, beauty supply outlets and department stores), or a *loofah* sponge brush made of natural bristles.

Five-Minute Skin Exercise

Moisten a complexion brush. Stroke over with soap or ordinary salad oil. Use a feathery rotary motion. Begin at the base of your throat. Work from your chin up to your ear level; then, move down to your nose and around your nostril wings. Keep up this feathery rotary motion. Work upward and finish on your forehead. Rinse with warm water, then with cool water. Rinse thoroughly, until you reach your hairline. *Pat,* do not rub, your face dry.

Benefits: The skin exercise helps coax pores into action, gives a natural boost to a sluggish circulation and helps the skin renew itself the natural way.

Tip: A loofah mitt (a coarse sponge) is available at many health stores and variety shoppes. Just slip it on your hand, like a mitt, and exercise your skin until your face glows. It reportedly helps smooth away lines, even diminishes the appearance of scars and has a natural way to correct the acidity of the skin. Use daily. The modern Orientals report that it helps remove the dead layers of the "scarfskin" or the surface skin, and acts as an elixir by revitalizing the nerve endings in the skin. This boosts skin activity to bring about a healthy, youthful appearance.

Fingertip Self-Massage Secret
of Oriental Royalists

The Oriental folk physicians, who were charged with the responsibility of keeping the royal family looking perpetually youthful, would regularly prescribe fingertip self-massage as a secret of regeneration. The benefit of self-massage is that the movement stimulates the "secret ingredient" of oxygen. The Orientalists reported that fingertip self-massage alerted circulation so that the bloodstream could then take up the oxygen to all skin cells and tissues, even to the tiniest and most remote corners of the body. When the skin cells were properly nourished with sufficient oxygen, then the skin was said to be able to thrive and glow with youthful health and vitality.

Five-Minute Self-Massage for Skin Awakening

Pull up the corners of your mouth and keep them up. Now, place the fingertips of both hands on your cheeks. Hold your cheek muscles tight. Now, slowly draw your mouth as far to the left as is comfortably possible; then go as far to the right as is comfortably possible. Be sure to keep your cheek muscles tight. Keep massaging your cheeks with your fingertips.

Note: Oriental folk physicians explained that merely pulling the mouth left and right would be of only minimal benefit. Instead, it is the *muscular* left and right pull, against the cheeks which you are massaging with your fingertips, that helps stimulate the needed oxygen flow and smooth out wrinkles. The Oriental physicians prescribed just five minutes daily (they kept approximate time, via an hour glass), and later reported that their royal patients were perpetually young through the divine grace of the gods.

How Orientals Use Simple
but Rejuvenating Water Treatments

Throughout the centuries, the Orientals have had few alternatives to cold ocean water for their cleansing needs. This may well have been a youth blessing in disguise, despite the apparent discomfort of taking a plunge in cold ocean water when one is generally sensitive to such temperatures. But the Orientals have been rewarded with silky smooth skin and luxuriant hair, which have given them the look of vitality even in their later years.

Today, the use of cold water is an Oriental secret for the look and feel of youth. Orientals often go to their health spas or follow this simple program at home:

Cold-Water Soak

Begin by taking a comfortably tepid bath to wash away dirt and grime. This also opens the pores. Now, splash comfortably cold water over the face and/or body. If you can attach a needle-shower head to your shower faucet, so much the better. Let the needle-shower spray your face, throat, arms and legs. The benefit here is that this cold needle-shower will perk up the bloodstream and send blood to these necessary regions, bearing tissue-feeding oxygen. Just ten minutes, as the Orientals prescribe, helps tighten up "aging" skin. You will emerge from the cold-water soak feeling as if you have just left the legendary Fountain of Youth. The Orientals think so, too.

Salt-Water Soak

The secret here is in the salt. Orientals explain that salt helps to attract moisture. It is essential to take a comfortably *warm* salt-water soak to open the pores and enable the salt to enter and remain within the skin pores. The salt then attracts and draws water — a sort of natural magnetic action. The water creates a balance from within that helps to fill up the tiny reservoirs located in the tissues. Once the reservoirs are filled with the water, they work to create a substitute fluid to take the place of diminishing natural fluids. This helps to retain moisture in the skin, ease away flaky and rough patches, and lubricate those tissues that might become fine lines of dryness. A unique benefit is that the salt attracts moisture that is compatible with the natural fluids of the skin. This natural moisture readily merges with existing liquids and helps boost the diminishing cellular levels so that the skin is encouraged to rejuvenate and reactivate its delicate equilibrium.

If you have ever envied the dew-fresh appearance of lovely Oriental complexions, you now know one of their secrets of helping to restore and retain youth-building moisture from within: simple salt-water soaking as often as possible.

Suggestion: Obtain sea salt or kelp from almost any health food store or special food shoppe. Add a handful to a tub of water, let the sea salt dissolve, and you have all the benefits of ocean bathing in the Orient, right in the privacy and convenience of your own home.

The Orientals have held that lackluster hair and aging skin occur whenever there is poor circulation. Therefore, they feel that the secret to youthful hair and skin is to stimulate sluggish circulation. In so doing, they feel that they can supercharge the body and mind to help promote the look and feel of youth. As living proof, we have the perpetually youthful appearance of Orientals. They have followed the secrets of their honored folk physicians and they have been rewarded with the youth of body and mind, the natural way.

SUMMARY:

1. Surrounded by oceans, the Orientals have tapped the briny depths for the secrets of perpetual youth. There are 16 Oriental secrets, used by Madge P. and others, that reportedly help rebuild and restore a youthful appearance.
2. A simple fruit, the lemon, can be used to promote the bloom of youth upon the skin and help restore a dew-fresh appearance for people of any age. A set of ten reported Oriental secrets show you the way.
3. An Oriental herbal face-lift helped smooth away Lena Z.'s wrinkles and furrows, making her look freshly young.
4. Orientals can exercise the skin for about five minutes and help improve the inner health of their bodies.
5. The fingertip self-massage secret of ancient Oriental royalists is now shared by many.
6. Cold-water soaks and salt-water soaks reportedly create a natural moisturization of the skin to rejuvenate the appearance.

11

The Hawaiian Fruits That Help Awaken and Rejuvenate the Digestive System

Fresh, raw fruits hold the secret of perpetual youthfulness for the healthy Hawaiians. For centuries, it has been traditional for these Pacific Islanders to turn to their abundance of luscious fruits for natural healing. Their legends are filled with the youth-building benefits to be found in many of the fresh, raw fruits that grow in the fertile soil of this paradise of the Pacific. Today, the secrets of some of these fruits are becoming known to many who have gone to Hawaii and discovered how the natural ingredients in these succulent plants have the ability to awaken and rejuvenate the digestive system. Once digestion is invigorated, healthy assimilation can be achieved. This helps to send a steady supply of essential vitamins, minerals, enzymes, amino acids and fatty acids throughout the body, working to build and rebuild the cells and tissues.

The forever-youthful health and apppearance of the native Hawaiians has become living proof of the secret rejuvenating ability of fresh raw fruits — the medicines of Nature, as prescribed by the traditional folk physicians of this garden of the Pacific.

How the Papaya is Used as a
Natural Fruit Medicine for Digestive Health

In the Hawaiian Islands, the papaya is hailed as the "melon of health" because it is used as a fruit medicine to help rejuvenate the digestive system. For this reason, the papaya is the popular breakfast fruit in Hawaii. Long ago, the natives were taught by Oriental folk physicians that this magical fruit possessed ingredients that alerted and reactivated the digestive system and, ever since, the papaya has been the Hawaiian way to natural, healthy digestion.

Melon-Like Fruit

What is the papaya? The fruit comes from a large, succulent, rapidly growing herbaceous plant; it is melon-like in its superficial characteristics. The skin is thin and smooth, and the papaya is green when unripe, but yellow-to-orange when ripe and ready for eating. The fruit may weigh a few ounces or as much as 25 pounds, depending upon the type.

The Hawaiians believe that eating the papaya for breakfast will help give them the strength of the young. In modern science, we have discovered that this folk-healing secret does have a valid basis.

Four Health Benefits of the Papaya Fruit

This luscious fruit of the Pacific contains these four health benefits:

1. Digestive Aid. Papaya has a youthfully vigorous papain enzyme, which helps promote digestive vigor; this will function in acidic, alkaline or neutral environment. The papain enzyme is said to be a miracle worker in helping to rejuvenate the body's digestion-assimilation process.

2. Respiratory Aid. Vitamins and minerals in the papaya work to help digest excessive sludge in the respiratory tract, ease coughing distress and promote more favorable throat and related breathing (oxygen) abilities. This helps boost better digestion since enzymes require a steady supply of needed oxygen.

3. Skin Aid. Papain, from the papaya, helps to dissolve the accumulation of secretions in the skin pores. Many Hawaiians will use a papaya peel as a "wash" over the skin. It helps wipe away infectious wastes, cleanse the grime-filled pores, improve better aeration of the body and thereby promote the look and feel of youthful skin.

4. Stomach Aid. Hawaiians have always looked to the papaya fruit as a natural medicine to help relax and soothe a troubled stomach. Papaya tea (a staple in the Islands, and now available in almost all health food stores) is especially soothing because it contains no caffeine or tannic acid, which often act as stomach irritants. Instead, papaya tea promotes a soothing enzymatic rhythm through its papain treasure.

The youthful vitality of the Hawaiians may well be their reward for adhering to folk tradition, which offers the luscious papaya as a natural medicine.

U.S. Government Praises the Health Values of the Papaya

The U. S. Department of Agriculture (Bulletin No. 77) has praised the papaya for its health values, by stating:

"It is well recognized that the papaya contains peculiar and valuable digestive properties which make it of great value in the diet. These peculiar digestive properties are largely due to the presence of papain, a very active ferment somewhat similar to pepsin. The papaya also ranks high as a source of vitamins, particularly A and C — vitamins associated, respectively, with growth and anti-scorbutic effects."

How Hawaiians Use Papaya

The U. S. Department of Agriculture adds, "In the tropics, the papaya is used for many purposes. Slices of green fruit rubbed over meat or boiled with tough meat are said to make the meat more tender. From the green fruit, an excellent stew, similar to the summer squash, is made."

Papaya Has a Treasure of Youth-Building Elements. Just one pound, an edible portion of papaya, will supply: 177 calories;

2.7 grams of protein; a miniscule 0.5 grams of fat; 45 energizing carbohydrate grams; 4 grams of bulk-forming fiber; 91 milligrams of nerve-building calcium; 73 milligrams of bone-strengthening phosphorus; 1.4 milligrams of blood-enriching iron; 7,945 units of skin-hair-eye revitalizing vitamin A; 14 milligrams of nerve-strengthening riboflavin; 18 milligrams of skin-respiratory improving riboflavin; 14 milligrams of hormone-feeding niacin; 254 milligrams of skin-tissue rejuvenating Vitamin C. Small wonder that Hawaiian and Pacific folk physicians have hailed the papaya as a natural medicine with amazing rejuvenating powers.

How Papaya Helped Rejuvenate an Executive

Business tensions churned the stomach of Glenn A. so that everything he ate felt like a lump in his abdomen. He sought to relieve this heaviness by taking one chemical medicine after another. Glenn A. would take medicines before eating with the hopes that they would boost his digestive powers; then he would take medicines after his meals, expecting them to help digest ingested food. It became a vicious cycle. When he took his chemical medicines, he experienced bloating and gaseous sensations. When he went without the chemical medicines, foods began to feel like a big blob in his stomach. Undoubtedly, tension and incorrect eating methods were responsible, but Glenn A. needed a more natural way to help rejuvenate his sluggish digestion.

Breakfast Papaya Produces Digestive Reactivation. At a convention held in Hawaii, he was given a plate of fresh papaya for breakfast. He was told that it was the secret of digestive youth among the Pacific Islanders. He scoffed, yet he ate the papaya (he did not take his medicine that morning); then he ate his regular breakfast. Within a matter of hours, he felt soothing digestion and a contentment that he thought belonged solely to young people. Noontime, he had more papaya as a "natural medicine" to be followed by his meal. In the evening, Glenn A. again had his papaya fruit as a digestive aid before the meal.

Benefits: The papaya enzyme is an organic substance, the

principal component of which is protein. Papaya enzymes work to change eaten food into particles, which can then be dissolved in body liquids and pass into the bloodstream. This helps to metabolize and assimilate the nutrients.

Once the enzymes from the Hawaiian "youth food" promoted digestive well-being and efficiency, Glenn A. felt relaxed, relieved and refreshed. He reportedly eats fresh papaya almost thrice daily now, and finds that this has rejuvenated his digestive system — the natural way.

How Papaya Juice Helps Create Intestinal Rejuvenation

Raw enzymes in fresh, raw papaya juice help to correct intestinal disorders within a reasonably short time. The juice contains valuable protein, natural citric, malic and tartaric acids, as well as potassium and phosphoric acids. These natural ingredients, when taken into an empty stomach, reportedly have a pronounced tonic effect upon the entire intestinal-digestive system. Many Hawaiians drink a glass of papaya juice every morning, and report that it regulates their body processes in a way that makes them feel as if they were growing younger throughout the day.

The Youth-Building Benefits of Papaya. Folk physicians report that papaya offers speedy relief for problems of gastritis, dyspepsia and digestive unrest. It works to attack and destroy decaying tissues in the system, and to cleanse the intestinal region of stored-up, decayed and infected wastes. The vitamins and minerals, as well as valuable enzyme proteins, work to stabilize normal body functions and nourish live tissues.

Modern native folk physicians prescribe the papaya as an antidote for disorders of the bowels and stomach. Papaya helps to ready food for metabolism, and by its action on protein, it helps form youth-building amino acids, which then work to help create a healthful acid-alkaline balance. The effectiveness of the papaya as a natural medicine against many disorders of the digestive-intestinal tract is attested to by those who, through consistent use, have received digestive harmony and overall healthy results.

How to Buy Papaya

Many health stores sell papaya as a raw fruit, or in bottled or canned form. If possible, try to obtain natural, organic papaya, which is yellow-to-orange in color, and handle it gently to avoid bruising. The ripe papaya fruit has a shelf life of only two days, so use it as soon as possible. To test for ripeness, be sure that the fruit is soft to the touch, but not mushy.

How to Use Papaya

Serve papaya as you would any melon or cantaloupe; you can flavor it with lemon or lime juice. It may also be served "a la carte," with seeds placed in the hollow. Papaya also makes an excellent fruit for a salad and combines well with most other fruits.

Papaya Punch: A Hawaiian natural fruit tonic is made this simple way: crush papaya pulp and thin it with orange juice; chill; drink this in the early morning.

Benefits: The rich supply of natural enzymes work to stir up sluggish digestion and create a soothing contentment in the region of the stomach. Hawaiians feel that the papaya punch gives them a rejuvenation boost and enables them to work with youthful gusto for most of the day.

How the Papaya Helps Tenderize Meats

Slices of the green fruit rubbed over meats or boiled together with tough meats are said to make them more tender. Those who have chewing problems should rub the papaya slices over meat to help increase its palatability. Many health stores sell powdered papaya for use as a natural meat tenderizer. The papain in the papaya fruit or papaya powder helps cause a slight pre-digestive action on tough connective tissues and fibers of meats, thus making the food easier to eat and digest.

Special Benefit: Papaya enzymes also have a splitting process on starches to make them more digestible; they also help digest fats. This combined action adds up to easier digestion and more enjoyable eating.

Banana — The Simple Fruit With Magic Rejuvenation Powers

Folk physicians of India and ancient Persia recommended the eating of bananas for "magic rejuvenation powers." It is reported that when Alexander the Great voyaged to these Eurasian countries in 327 B.C., he found the inhabitants eating bananas to help ward off evil spirits and bring about the feelings of youth. Many Orientals regarded this golden fruit as Nature's secret of perpetual youth. To this day, bananas are known for promoting healthy digestion and helping to create the look and feel of youth.

Youthful Energy, Better Digestion, Cellular Rejuvenation

In a reported situation, doctors were able to boost youthful energy, better digestion and a form of cellular rejuvenation by prescribing bananas to ailing patients.[1] These patients reportedly had chronic intestinal indigestion, "aging" metabolism and other symptoms of tissue depletion. When given whole, fresh bananas, the patients began to recover.

Benefits: Bananas help promote the retention of calcium, phosphorus and nitrogen, which then work to build sound and youthfully regenerated tissues. Bananas also contain invert sugar, which is an aid to youthful metabolism. This "magic" fruit creates an alkalizing action on intestinal contents and offers soft banana fiber and the bulky residue provided by pectins. By re-establishing the delicate yin-yang balance in the digestive system, nutrients can be better assimilated, and this can serve to improve digestion and bring about cellular rejuvenation.

How a Simple, All-Natural Program Boosts Youthful Health

In the previously mentioned case, the doctors sought to put their patients on an all-natural youth-restorative program. They

---

[1] Haas, S.V., and Haas, M.P.: *Postgraduate Medicine* 7:239.

were told to eat bananas regularly, and certain other foods were excluded from the diet.

Forbidden foods: Any cereal grain such as corn, wheat, bread, cake, toast, crackers or breakfast cereals; sugar was taboo, either as sweetening or in the form of candy, pastries, breads or corn syrups, and milk was not allowed.

Results: This all-natural program was a modified controlled-fasting regimen used in the Orient for centuries. The bananas were able to perform their healing rejuvenation without the interference of offending foods. The patients recovered, while eating as many as ten bananas a day and excluding the previously mentioned foods. They looked and felt youthful — they had tapped the magic banana secret of the Orient!

Secret Oriental Banana Prescription

The ancient folk physicians had their ways of determining how natural fruit medicines could produce a feeling of youthful well-being. Enlightened royal physicians also had a secret prescription for helping to perpetuate the youth and health of their imperial rulers. They would prescribe the eating of bananas with non-starch vegetables and other fruits, but *not with acid fruits* (oranges or tangerines) and *never with starches or proteins*. (Note that in the previously mentioned program, prescribed by a modern doctor, the forbidden foods were high-starch and modified-protein, such as milk. We can see that the ancient folk physicians were well ahead of their time in knowing that bananas often generate more rejuvenating benefits when metabolized without the interference of starches or proteins.)

Throughout the modern Orient, many folks will eat bananas alone or go on a one-day banana fast to help heal their digestive disturbances and enjoy the rewards of youthfully healthful living.

Banana: The Golden Treasure of Youth

The velvety smooth banana offers a golden treasure of health. It has an alkaline reaction in the system and is a prime source of calcium, phosphorus, manganese, vitamin A, pyridoxine, inositol, folic acid, vitamin C and many more nutrients. These work to help maintain the health of the skin, eyes and mucous membranes, and to detoxify infectious bacteria, aid in the body's protein storage, build resistance to allergies, relieve constipation, soothe and heal colitis and ulcers, soothe the kidneys, boost the appetite via nourishment of the taste buds and create a well-balanced, youthful digestive system. The Orientals hailed the banana as a magic fruit of the gods. Now, we may all taste of this magic fruit and enjoy better health.

The Apple: Secret Youth Fruit of the Hawaiians

The smooth complexions of the Hawaiians and Polynesians, their forever-young athletic movements, happy laughter and effervescent energy may well be traced to another "secret youth fruit." Almost every Polynesian includes the apple in his daily eating plan, and here are some of the reported benefits:

For Upset Stomach, Eat an Apple

This folk prescription has worked wonders in restoring youthful digestive functions to Hawaiians and Polynesians of all ages. Today, modern Hawaiians still cling to this secret youth fruit and enjoy a youthful digestive system.

Modern Benefit: The scientific basis for this is that the active medicinal principle of the apple is *pectin,* a natural therapeutic ingredient found in the inner portion of the rinds or in the apple pomace. Its restorative power lies in its protective coating action by virtue of its ability to act as an absorbent and demulcent. Pectin aids in detoxification by supplying the galacturonic acid needed for the elimination of certain noxious substances. Pectin also helps to prevent putrefaction of protein matter in the alimentary canal.

True, the Polynesian and Pacific folk physicians did not have this scientific interpretation at hand, but they did have wisdom and knowledge. When they saw that a natural fruit promoted digestive rejuvenation, they prescribed it to their patients. It worked then, and many people are finding that it works today.

Polynesian Digestive Tonic

Edna N., a victim of digestive turbulence ever since her youth, suffered the distress of colitis and irregularity even when she took a vacation in the paradise of the Pacific. Her Oriental tour director was disturbed by the fact that Edna N. was wasting her expensive vacation in her room. He recommended a Polynesian folk remedy that reportedly could heal Edna's "senile stomach," as she called it.

How to Make a Polynesian Digestive Tonic: Simmer apple parings in boiled milk for up to 15 minutes. Then drink one warm cup every hour until relief is felt.

Feels Young All Over. Desperate for relief, Edna N. tried this Polynesian digestive tonic. It took up to five hours for relief to be felt, but by nightfall, Edna N. was so relieved from her digestive unrest that she said she felt "young all over," thanks to her Oriental tour director's secret.

Benefits: The simmering brings out the ingredients in the apple so they can combine with the buffering alkalinity of the calcium in the milk. This creates a mild acidity, which acts as an intestinal germicide or inhibitant, thus restraining the excessive amount of the putrefactive organisms responsible for digestive "senility." The malic acid in the Polynesian digestive tonic acts as a diuretic, so that its action on the kidneys can promote urinary excretion and, hence, the elimination of toxic wastes. This secret may well be the greatest value of this Oriental digestive rejuvenation tonic.

How Apples Help Correct Problems of Anemia

The remarkably low incidence of anemia among the rich-blooded Polynesians may well be due to their daily eating of whole, fresh apples. The folk physicians of the Pacific have long prescribed apples to "warm the blood" and to put "color and the bloom of youth in the cheeks." This is more than just folklore medicine. Today, we know that the natural acid content of apples aid the body in absorbing iron from food. Combined with the fructose (natural fruit sugar) in apples, the fruit helps metabolize and assimilate iron, which is then used by the blood cells for youthful enrichment and regeneration. The apple has always been considered a "blood building" food by the Polynesians. They knew that a rich, red bloodstream began with better digestion, and that the apple's nutrients can be part of this healthful internal rhythm.

The Pineapple — Miracle Fruit of
Youthful Digestion

This miracle fruit, which at one time may have been the staple food of the pioneering Polynesians, contains *bromelain,* a "magic enzyme" that helps in the digestion and assimilation of nutrients.

To the Polynesians, eating several slices of fresh pineapple, or drinking a cup of freshly prepared pineapple juice, is a pre-dinner digestive aid. The folk physicians pointed out that if the Polynesians wanted to eat and enjoy food with the gustatory pleasure of a young warrior, it would be well for them to begin *and* end their meals with pineapple slices.

Secret Benefit: The *bromelain* enzyme in the pineapple helps to prevent the body fluids from becoming too acidic or too alkaline, again, a principle in maintaining the precious yin-yang balance. Furthermore, the bromelain enzyme is able to combine with and neutralize either acidic or alkaline substances. Bromelain is the raw material from which most of the hormones are made, and this enzyme also works to help the liver produce a protein known as albumin, which establishes detoxification. The bromelain enzyme helps body fluids wash off waste materials to cleanse the kidneys and related digestive organs. So we can see that the *bromelain* enzyme found in the mellow, yellow golden pineapple may well hold one of the keys to better digestion.

Do as the Polynesians Do

Adhering to the advice of the ancient Oriental folk physicians, the modern Polynesians still believe that digestive rejuvenation is possible through beginning and ending their meals with pineapple slices or fresh pineapple juices. This sends forth a valuable supply of vitamins, minerals and youth-building enzymes to help maintain a healthy digestive system.

The Melon — Nature's Secret Digestive Aid

The melon is a soft, juicy, tasty fruit; but to the Hawaiians, it is also a valuable digestive aid. Island tradition points to the healing of stomachache, constipation and "weak" digestion through the simple eating of the melon.

Throughout the South Pacific, the hardy and youthful Islanders enjoy such digestion-improving fruits as the cantaloupe, casaba melon, Persian melon, honeydew and watermelon.

Secret Benefit: The melon contains vitamins A and C, which help rejuvenate internal and external skin tissues. In particular, Vitamin C produces collagen, a natural cementing material that holds body cells together, helps firm up the walls of the blood vessels in the digestive system and helps in healing worn-out and wasted cells and tissues.

Benefits: The fibrous structure of many raw melons provides two unique physical benefits. (1) The chewing process exercises the muscles of the face and jaw. (2) This forces the food over the teeth and soft tissues. It then creates a "detergent" action in the mouth, and cleanses the saliva so that it helps to detoxify harmful bacteria that may be lodged within the oral crevices. This sends a supply of well-washed liquid into the throat and digestive system — a natural process which the Polynesians discovered centuries ago.

Hawaiians prefer vine-ripened melons. The benefit here is that as the melon *naturally* ripens its fructose content increases, thus giving it better taste and a sweeter juice. Also, the ripening process increases the effectiveness of the supply of vitamins and minerals, making them more beneficial to the digestive system.

Although the ancient Polynesian folk physicians did not have such scientific knowledge at their disposal, they did possess wisdom and awareness. They saw that melons promoted youthful digestion and recognized this as a magic sign of health. They prescribed melons for helping to prolong the prime of youth, and the well-known, vigorous youth of Hawaiians, even in their later years, attests to the fact that fruits offer a golden key to the doorway of better youth and health.

Health-Boosting Benefits of Hawaiian Fruits

Fresh Fruits from the Pacific offer a horn of plenty insofar as health-boosting benefits are concerned. For example:

Fruits Boost Natural Acids. Hydrochloric acids aid in the digestion of protein and fat. Hawaiian fruits (sold at almost all markets) help produce natural hydrochloric acid in the "aging" system.

Fruits aid in *Self-Cleansing.* Natural fruit acid inhibits the growth of the germs of putrefacation and, thus, provides a self-cleansing action.

Fruits Supply Bulk. Hawaiian fruit pulp supplies bulk to stimulate peristalsis, the waves of motion in the digestive tract that help move the food mass through the system. This helps prevent constipation. Fruit juice is a wholesome, predigested food, which was prescribed by Oriental-Polynesian folk physicians as being of medicinal value in restoring regularity.

Fruits Improve Protein Metabolism. Fruit juices (especially from the pineapple) contain properties that aid protein digestion. For example, these fruit juices help digest the albumin in eggs to convert it into a liquid. Such fruit juices work upon tough protein to break it down into usable and youth-building amino acids.

How to Ease the Urge for Tobacco or Alcohol

Modern Hawaiian folk physicians explain that fresh fruits (and their juices) help create a distaste for tobacco or alcohol. Nutrients in the fruit work to dilate the blood vessels and open up the capillaries to prevent obstruction. This counteracts the tobacco-alcohol craving, which has been traced to a tightening of the vessels and nerve networks in the body. Many modern physicians agree that fresh fruits and fruit juices do help control the psycho-physiological urge to partake of these unhealthy substances.

The people of the Polynesian islands in the Pacific have traditionally held that fruits will help awaken and rejuvenate the digestive system. The Hawaiians, themselves, are living proof of the healing powers of fresh fruits and fresh fruit juices. Today, you can help promote better digestion and help yourself look and fell as young as the healthy Hawaiians with simple — but effective — fruit medicines!

HIGHLIGHTS:

1. The papaya is used as a natural fruit medicine by the Hawaiians. It offers four basic health benefits, which helped to free Glenn A. from his nervous stomach and chemical-medicine addiction.

2. The golden banana is an Oriental secret of youthful energy, better digestion and cellular rejuvenation. The secret Oriental banana prescription is a Hawaiian way to better digestive vigor.

3. The apple is a Hawaiian "youth-fruit." A Polynesian digestive tonic helped Edna N. enjoy youthful regularity and freedom from years of internal upheaval.

4. Enzymes in the pineapple promote overall revitalization through the improvement of the digestive system.

5. Vine-ripened melons offer a treasure of digestive rejuvenation. Hawaiian folk physicians hail the melon as a valuable key to perpetual youth.

12

The Miracle Vegetable Protein from the Orient — A Key to Forever-Young Vitality

For thousands of years, soybeans have been a valuable source of nutrition throughout the Far East. This simple, nourishing vegetable protein food, grown easily on most soils and in most climates, has served to nourish, invigorate and rejuvenate the health of the Orientals. In regions where the soybean has, at times, been the only available food, it has been able to provide all the known nutritional elements to maintain health and vitality.

Soybeans — A Meatless Source of Complete Protein

The secret of the youth-building power of soybeans may well be in their endowment of all the essential amino acids (forms of protein) in good proportions. While most fruits, vegetables and grains do contain amino acids, they lack or are deficient in one or more of the essential youth-building substances. Soybeans, on the other hand, contain *all* the essential amino acids that work to build and rebuild good health. The Orientals were wise to note that eating soybeans when other foods were unavailable helped give them vigor, vitality and a feeling of youthful health. In recent years, it has been discovered that

153

the complete amino acid pattern of this meatless protein has been a great factor in the healthful lives of the Orientals.

Soybeans — Meat Without a Bone

That's what millions of Orientals call this high-protein food. They have recognized the fact that this little legume (bean) is about the only vegetable that can effectively take the place of meat. So highly have Orientals regarded soybeans that battles once raged over the Manchurian fields where the top-quality soybeans have always grown. Throughout the centuries, the "meat without a bone" has become a miracle vegetable protein that has given the Orientals "forever-young" vitality — something that traditional meat eaters may not have experienced. Today, many have tapped the secret of Oriental health — the traditional eating of soybeans.

The Magic Ingredient in Soybeans That Helps Promote Perpetual Youth

The Chinese and Japanese often enjoy youthful living well beyond the "century mark." It is important to note that in their diet — so poor by Western standards — the soybean has been the foundation. During periods of privation and famine, the Orientals have cultivated soybeans, which have sustained them and kept them healthy and perpetually young. The Orientals call the soybean a "holy bean," and will look to it as a substitute for meat, dairy, eggs and other grains. The know that soybeans do more than just keep them alive; they have "magic ingredients" that give people a feeling of added endurance, youthful vitality and surprisingly youthful appearance. Modern researchers have tapped the secret of the soybean and come up with its youth-building "magic ingredient" — *lecithin.*

Secret Youth Power of Soybean's Lecithin

Lecithin is a natural emulsifier of the fats in the body. It plays a decisive youth-building role in stimulating metabolism throughout all the cells and tissues of the body. It nourishes the brain and nerve cells, and is involved in the nucleus of *all* body cells.

The Magic Power of Lecithin: This ingredient in soybeans has a magic-like power as a phospholipid (fat-dissolving agent), and helps metabolize fat and send nutrients to the brain, heart, muscles, bone marrow, liver, kidneys and spinal cord. Lecithin is also present in the endocrine glands and the nervous system, and is chiefly responsible for hormone manufacture. Hormones hold the secret of perpetual youth, and lecithin is the spark that ignites the flow of body hormones.

The Ten Youth-Building Powers of Lecithin in Soybeans

Lecithin works to create the following ten youth-building powers:

1. Helps to metabolize fat accumulations and dissolve thick deposits of excess cholesterol.
2. Works via the endocrine-nervous-circulatory systems to help regulate a normal basal metabolic rate.
3. Enters into the regeneration of tissues and cells to help repair breakage and promote better muscular strength.
4. Works on the motor nerves of the body to create youthful fitness in the functions of strength, agility and flexibility.
5. Enters into the oxygen intake capacity, which enables you to work better and to enjoy better energy.
6. Strengthens the respiratory reserves, which helps improve your ventilatory capacity. Better aeration of the body means better circulation.
7. A better metabolic process and distribution of amino acids enables lecithin to build resistance to ligamentous injuries and strengthen resistance to strains in the spine, shoulders and knees.
8. Helps regulate blood cholesterol and blood pressure levels, and also adjusts the peripheral levels.
9. Enters into the arterial-neuron structures, building resistance to problems associated with arteriosclerosis.
10. Influences better mineral absorption to help strengthen the bones and skeleton to resist against the problems of osteoporosis, or brittle bones.

The enviable youth of the Oriental may well be traced to this "magic ingredient" in soybeans. Soybeans are available at almost every corner market or shopping center, as well as almost all health food shoppes.

Soybeans for Better Energy, Improved Memory, Steady Hands

Soybean lecithin helped an 88-year old researcher enjoy better energy and youthful health. Edward R. Hewitt[1] wrote:

"Lecithin is well known to have a very great emulsifying action on fats. It is reasonable to suppose that it would have the same emulsifying action in the body . . . With older people, the fats remain high in the blood for from 5 to 7 hours, and in some cases as long as 20 hours, thus giving the fats more time to become located in the tissues. If lecithin is given to older people before a fatty meal it has been found that the fats in the blood return to normal in a short time, in the same way they do in younger people . . .

"I myself also have observed that my memory is better than it was before I took lecithin regularly. My nervous reactions are still perfectly normal at 88. My hands are much steadier than those of any doctor who tested me."

Secret Ingredient: Soybeans offer a special type of lecithin, *unlike lecithin found in other foods.* Soybean lecithin contains a treasure of *auxines,* identified as "vegetable hormones," which nourish and replenish the glandular system and help them pour forth youth-building hormones.

Why Orientals Call Soybeans Their "Perfect Food"

Orientals traditionally call soybeans their "perfect food" because it has a rich treasure of these nutrients: *Protein* (of which up to 94% is digested and well-utilized by the body, and containing *all* essential amino acids); *vegetable fat,* which is healthfully nourishing; *calcium and phosphorus,* for the skeletal-nerve system; *iron,* to enrich the bloodstream; *potassium,* to maintain blood-nerve balance; *vitamin A,* to nourish the eyes

---

[1]Edward R. Hewitt, *The Years Between 75 and 90.* (Health Publishing Co., San Francisco, Calif., 1957).

and skin and act as carrier of other nutrients; *vitamin C,* to help build and rebuild cells and tissues; *B-complex vitamins,* for the nervous and respiratory systems; *vitamin K,* to help assist in blood coagulation; *vitamin E,* which is needed to rejuvenate the heart muscle and maintain better oxygen consumption.

Soybeans offer more potassium than just about any other food, and they have the top-notch source of pantothenic acid (B-complex vitamin for the nervous system). Also, the iron in soybeans is 96% digestible, in contrast to most iron foods, such as meats, which are not well-assimilated by the body. Soybean oil is 51.5% linoleic acid (an essential fatty acid that helps emulsify blood cholesterol to build resistance against the formation of cholesterol deposits). All these elements are found in healthful abundance in this Oriental "perfect food," which has served as a staple food in the Orient for thousands of years.

How Soybeans Gave Rose B. the Look and Feel of Youth

Saleswoman Rose B. found the hours stretching endlessly as she worked on the main floor of a department store. She felt a heavy pressure between her shoulder blades that caused her to walk with a stooped gait. She suffered from such indigestion that she subsisted on a diet of dry toast, black coffee and chain-smoking of cigarettes. Whatever she ate would cause acid upset, and she experienced varying degrees of colitis. She felt a stiffening of her fingers, her skin was pale and her hair was stringy. Her memory was fuzzy and she looked and felt much older than her middle 40's. Even when she took a reduction in working time (and a reduction in pay), she found the lighter schedule just as intolerable as the full time schedule. Rose B. had become a dismal picture of declining health.

A Customer-Friend Offers Rose B. an Oriental Soybean Secret. A customer-friend inquired about Rose's absence from the store and was told that the saleswoman was "feeling low " The friend returned when Rose was in the store and, expressing concern over Rose's fading health, she told Rose of her recent trip to the Orient. She noted that the Chinese and Japanese, as well as the Pacific Islanders, exhibited youthful agility even in old age. She said that the Orientals look to soybeans as the secret of rejuvenation and told Rose B. to try eating soybeans to improve her health. Rose B. had little to lose. She began to eat soybeans regularly. Here is how soybeans helped improve her health.

Soybeans Offer Digestive Balance. The high alkalinity of soybeans (reportedly some 20 times more alkaline than milk) created a healthful acid-alkaline balance and eased the distress of burning stomach acid. This was the familiar yin-yang principle of celestial harmony within the body — thanks to soybeans.

Soybeans Improve Skin and Hair Health. The rich treasure of vitamins and youth-building minerals worked to feed the bloodstream, enriching the health of the skin and hair. Rose B. looked better as her skin complexion improved and became dew-fresh; her hair became naturally shiny and her scalp became free of dandruff flakes.

Soybeans Improve the Posture and Finger Flexibility. The combination of essential amino acids as well as the supply of phospholipids promoted a nourishment of the skeletal structure and also helped regulate the cholesterol levels. This helped improve Rose's posture and gave more flexibility to her stiff fingers and joints.

Soybeans Help Create a Youthful Feeling Internally and Externally. Internally, the rich supply of lecithin helped create better fat distribution within her body. Externally, the linoleic acid and linolenic acids (both are unsaturated fatty acids) helped to promote healthy tissues, cells, skin and scalp. The carefully Nature-created balance of ingredients worked in *harmony* within Rose B. to create a youthful feeling — inside and out.

Thanks to soybeans, and a better living program that called for the elimination of tobacco and caffeine-containing coffee and tea, Rose B. could now walk with the youthful posture and vigorous energy typical of the sturdy, soybean-eating Orientals.

How Cooked Soybeans Offer
Protein-Plus Health Benefits

Nature has decreed that soybeans must be cooked in order to be eaten. There is wisdom in this natural law of healthful eating, for soybeans contain all essential amino acids, but three of them — lysine, methionine and trypsin — are enhanced by cooking. This creates a better amino acid balance than that derived from meat.

Here's how it works: The soybean is the one food that offers "protein plus" through cooking. The biological benefits of protein are related to the quantity of any essential amino acids made available from the protein. Soy protein has *lysine,* which is heat-sensitive when exposed to temperatures even as low as those used for milk pasteurization (148°-150°F.)

Increased heat and extended cooking time reduces the amount of lysine available in most foods. However, soybeans also contain *methionine,* another amino acid that acts as a limiting factor to help seal in the valuable lysine during the heating.

The third amino acid, *trypsin,* acts as an inhibitor (trypsin helps your enzymes digest protein) that cooperates in the biological pattern so that during the heating of the soybean, all amino acids maintain a unique and health-building balance. It is this balance that stems from the ancient Oriental law of healthful living, namely, the yin-yang balance, which helps build better health of the body and mind at all ages. The soybean appears to be such a balanced food, insofar as amino acid metabolism is concerned.

Benefits: The well-balanced level of high-grade, biologically complete protein in the soybean is the foundation for physical fitness, vigor and better insulation against illness. As living proof, we can look to the hardy Orientals who have subsisted upon soybeans (frequently, as their sole source of nourishment except for water) and enjoyed robust health and youthful vitality even in old age. The soybean deserves its name — the "holy bean."

How to Prepare Soybeans

Obtain good quality soybeans from any large food market or corner produce store. If possible, obtain organically grown soybeans from your nearest health store or organic produce outlet. Wash the soybeans under free-flowing cold tap water and place a desired amount in a kettle. Fill with water until the kettle is about three-quarters full. Let this stand overnight. *Note:* This overnight soaking softens the beans; they will also swell up to almost double in bulk, so be certain there is enough room in your kettle.

The next day, boil the soybeans in the same water. Boil until the soybeans are soft, usually 2-1/2 to 4 hours. When ready, eat the soybeans and use the liquid as a sauce. This liquid is an excellent source of all-natural vitamins and minerals. Orientals traditionally use the liquid either as a sauce *or as a beverage.* When comfortably hot, it can be an excellent *soybean tea —* the *only* tea that has a top-notch supply of well-balanced, biologically complete protein. Flavor with herbs, vegetized seasoning or sea salt, if desired.

Soybeans Offer Vitality-Boosting Nutrients

The Orientals have praised soybeans, more than any other vegetable, for offering such vitality-boosting nutrients. The reason is that soybeans differ from most beans in that they contain triple the amount of *protein,* a small amount of sugar, but *no starch.* This makes soybeans an excellent food for calorie-watchers. Soybeans supply biologically balanced, essential amino acids, nerve and bone-building calcium and nearly all known vitamins. It is this interrelationship of so many nutrients that helps boost life, health and youthful vitality.

For Health-Plus, Try Soybean Flour

It is said that one tablespoon of soybean flour offers almost the same food value as an egg. Most large food stores and health shoppes sell soybean flour. It can be used to make muffins, breads, pancakes or biscuits. *Tip:* Make morning pancakes or waffles with soybean flour and get a terrific "protein boost" at the start of the day. For a high-protein breakfast, soybean flour pancakes or waffles are powerhouses of vital youth.

The Oriental Way to Make Soybean Milk

Three times a day, Joseph K. drinks "vegetable milk." Joseph K. shares many an adult's dislike of cow's milk, and he also suffers from allergic rhinitis and bronchial upsets, which are often the results of drinking cow's milk. This may be a psychosomatic rejection of cow's milk, forced upon him as a youngster; nevertheless, he has found that the Oriental secret of "vegetable milk" helps give him a tremendous boost of vitality and energy. Here's how he makes it:

Vegetable Milk: Soak 1 cup of soybeans in 3 cups of water for up to 48 hours. Pour off the water and set it aside for future use as a sauce for vegetables. Now grind the soaked soybeans through a meat chopper or put them in a blender and chop very fine. Add up to 6 cups of freshly poured water to the soybeans in a kettle. Boil for 30 minutes; then strain through cheesecloth or a fine colander. (If desired, season with sea salt and a little organic honey.) You now have "vegetable milk" (the portion strained through the cheesecloth). Save the mashed soybean pulp as a vegetable side dish. You may drink the milk just as you do cow's milk.

Joseph K. finds that this milk gives him pep and energy, a storehouse of protein and relatively few calories in comparison with cow's milk. Most important, he develops no allergic symptoms. This Oriental secret of "vegetable milk" has made him feel healthy and invigorated.

Why Orientals Value Soybean
Protein Above Meat Protein

Modern Oriental scientists and researchers still value soybean protein above meat protein. The reason is that the *complete* protein present within soybeans is more beneficial than incomplete or fragmentary proteins present in meats. Modern Orientals note that if just *one* essential amino acid is partially missing (as in meats, fish, eggs or grains), the result is that all the remaining amino acids are reduced in the same proportion. Consequently, the body receives less available protein for its use. In other words, one amino acid complements the other.

In soybeans, the presence of *all* amino acids means that the body is able to have a high level of protein synthesis. The biological value of soybean protein is extremely high; this means that soybeans offer a high proportion of the protein that can be absorbed by the enzymatic digestive tract and made available for body regeneration.

Meat Protein May Be Less Effective

Meat protein may be weak or deficient in one or more amino acids. Consequently, the protein metabolic core in the cell will use some of the amino acids but release the rest from the body as fuel, as if they were lowly carbohydrates. Oriental physicians of today also note that soybean protein is better absorbed and assimilated by the digestive tract. Nature has made this so by giving it a well-balanced supply of amino acids. In modern interpretation, we look to the inviolate decree of Nature: *the whole is greater than the sum of its parts.*

The robust good health of the Oriental may well be traced to his discovery of soybeans as a source of biologically complete vegetable proteins. Soybeans, in contrast to meat, contain no hard fats, no high calories, no pound-building starch, no cholesterol-forming ingredients, little uric acid formatives, no chemicals such as those injected into livestock and no infectious animal diseases. Soybeans may well be the Oriental secret of "forever-young" vitality. They have nourished the Orientals for thousands of years, without subjecting them to the diseases of Western civilization. Today, soybeans are considered miracles from the Orient — and they are available at your corner food market.

MAIN POINTS:

1. The soybean is the "miracle vegetable protein" of the Orient. A complete protein, it offers biologically balanced amino acids for better health.
2. Soybeans offer a "magic ingredient" called lecithin, which helps promote perpetual youth. A set of ten youth-building benefits are made available by this Oriental food.
3. Soybeans helped an 88-year old man enjoy better energy, steady hands and an improved memory. A "secret in-

gredient" is *auxine,* a "vegetable hormone," which helps promote rejuvenation through replenishment within the glandular system.

4. Orientals call the soybean the "perfect food" for its rich treasure of nutrients in a delicate balance rarely found in other foods.

5. Rose B. was restored to the look and feel of youth and enjoyed freedom from indigestion and premature aging through a natural health program featuring soybeans.

6. Cooked soybeans offer three special youth-building amino acids that may be the "secret" of Oriental youthfulness.

7. For "vegetable milk," try Joseph K.'s easy method. It helped him find freedom from allergies and distress.

8. Soybeans are valued for protein power above that of meat protein.

13

Oriental Secrets of Toning the Heart for Youth and Health

The long-living and youthful Orientals have tapped the secrets of how to keep the heart young and healthy, and they have been rewarded with amazingly low incidences of arteriosclerosis and related heart diseases. Traditionally, the Orientals have looked to the plants of the fields and the fish of the ocean for their nourishment and good health. They have discovered that by eating the "right" kind of fat, they not only nourish their bodies but provide youthful "oil" for their hearts. The result is that right up to our modern times, the heart-attack rate for the Orientals is extremely low in comparison to the high heart attack rate for the Western world.

The Orientals have learned that oils from plants and fish can have a beneficial effect upon their hearts, providing them with resistance to cardiac difficulties such as those that often afflict Westerners who eat excessive fats from animal sources. The Orientals enjoy forever-young hearts in advanced age because of their awareness of the values of plant and fish oils. Today, Westerners are slowly discovering the Oriental secrets and reaping the benefits of better youth and health, beginning with the heart — the "heart" of long life and health.

How Orientals Rejuvenate Their Hearts
With Plant or Fish Oils

It is traditional for Orientals to use as many plant or fish oils as possible. They are aware that these beneficial oils are free of cholesterol (found in fats from animal sources). Cholesterol is a porridge-like substance, which can become a fatty deposit that thickens the artery walls. This reduces the amount of space in the arteries for the blood to circulate. If this happens in the large arteries that send nourishing blood into the heart, it can cause an obstruction, which can lead to a heart attack. Although the ancient Orientals may not have been aware of our modern scientific findings, they had the folk wisdom to realize that the use of plant or fish oils provided good health for the heart.

Plant or fish oils are prime sources of unsaturated fatty acids, which combine with other substances within the body to help carry such essential ingredients as linolenic, linoleic and arachidonic acids through the miles of blood vessels, thus helping to cleanse away sludge and obstructions. The unsaturated fatty acids in plant or fish oils have this secret benefit: they work to keep cholesterol on the move. These oils contain pyridoxine, one of the B-complex vitamins, which acts as an energizer or starter to help pump the unsaturated fatty acids through the blood vessels and arteries so they can perform their self-cleansing tasks. This helps lubricate and elasticize the arterio-network so it can send healthful oxygen-bearing blood to the heart.

How the Right Kind of "Oriental Fat"
Helped Give Paul L. a New Lease on His Heart

Factory foreman Paul L. always ate with gusto. Believing that his hard work required him to eat heavily, he would fill himself up on high animal-fatty foods such as sausage, poultry (with the skin), thick gravies, thickly buttered sandwiches, heavy cream soups, and snacks of potato chips and pizza.

Paul L. felt recurring chest pains and breathing difficulties, yet he refused to believe that his heavy fat diet had anything to do with it. He insisted that his hard work necessitated a corresponding "hard" diet.

Visiting Orientals Give Him the Secret of Heart Health. As part of an economic business exchange, a group of Oriental factory supervisors came to Paul's plant to learn about American business methods. Paul L. escorted several of the visitors throughout the industrial complex, after which they had dinner in the company commissary.

Paul L. ordered a thick slice of fat-covered meat, swimming in heavy gravy, as well as several cold cuts. He also had thick slices of bleached white bread with generous amounts of salty butter. He noted that the slim, trim and youthful Orientals preferred a meal of lean fish, raw vegetables, and skim milk pudding, all of which were on the menu. The Orientals said that this food program gave them the strength and energy of youth, and they smilingly admitted to being over the age of fifty. They were lean and agile, yet could put in a full ten-hour work schedule in their factories in the Orient.

In contrast, Paul L. found his days growing more wearisome, his breathing more difficult and his senses more blurred. He was told by the Orientals that modern Asiatics adhere to the health secrets of their ancestral folk physicians and that they emphasize "healthy fats" from plants and fish. This combination of ancient and modern health programs, to help give vital energy to the heart, was recommended to Paul L. by the Oriental visitors. Here are the results:

Enjoys Bounce Back to Youthful Health. Within three weeks of a healthful Oriental-based food program, Paul L. found that his chest pains subsided, his breathing became easier, his senses became youthfully sharp. More important, he could compete with the physical stamina of the younger men in the plant. Paul L. had bounced back to youthful health.

The Oriental Way to Better Heart Health

The modern Orientals know that fat is necessary; yet they say that there are "right" fats and "wrong" fats. This knowledge is a combination of secrets from Oriental folk physicians throughout the past centuries and modern discoveries on how to feed the heart to give it youthful vitality. The low incidence of heart distress in the Orient may well be living proof of the benefits of this Oriental way to better heart health.

"Right" Fats

These are the polyunsaturated fats, or those that tend to lower the level of blood cholesterol. These include: modern-day dietetic margarines; all vegetable oils; all fish oils; poultry (without the skin); nuts; whole-grain bread and non-processed cereals; fruits; lean meats; uncreamed cottage cheese; skim milk; peanut butter; all vegetables; low-fat desserts such as gelatin and sherbet.

"Wrong" Fats

These are the saturated fats, or those that tend to raise the level of blood cholesterol. These include: butter; fatty meats; luncheon meats; whole milk; most cheeses made from whole milk; eggs; chocolate; lard; thick gravies; cream; coconut; desserts and pastries made with animal fats such as lard or butter; shellfish; creamed foods.

Fat Differences

Polyunsaturated fats are those that tend to be liquid at room temperature; they are present in good amounts in liquid vegetable, seed and fish oils. Saturated fats are those that raise the cholesterol level and are generally of animal origin and are solid at room temperature.

The "Right" Fats, Which Orientals Eat for Better Heart Health. These are the "right" fats that Orientals favor as a means of helping to keep their hearts and bodies in a feeling of youthful health:

Lean beef; veal or lamb; fish; chicken and turkey; all fruits and vegetables; nuts — raw, oil or dry-roasted; modern dietetic margarine; skim milk; uncreamed cottage cheese; vegetable oils; dietetic mayonnaise and salad dressings; whole-grain breads; unbleached macaroni and spaghetti; whole-grain cereals; natural brown rice; puddings made with skim milk; gelatin desserts; sherbet; angel food cake; peanut butter; jams and jellies made without sugar.

The "Wrong" Fats, Which Orientals Avoid. These are the "wrong"fats, which Orientals say should be limited as a means of helping to keep down the formation of excess cholesterol, which is known to be injurious to the heart and general health:

Pork; bacon; spareribs; sausage; prepared meats; gravies; poultry skin; avocados; coconut; olives; butter; whole and canned milk; cream; most cheeses made from whole milk; cream soups; cakes; cookies; doughnuts; griddle cakes; biscuits; pastries; whipped cream desserts; chocolate; ice cream; pie crusts; fried foods; potato chips; creamed foods; products made with lard or hydrogenated shortenings.

Oriental Secret: Orientals limit or restrict their use of egg yolk, kidney and brains, which they say are among the "wrong" fat foods. Today, we know that these are extremely high in cholesterol and an excess may be harmful to the heart. Orientals have known this "secret" for many generations. Today, they follow the health rules of their ancestors and enjoy enviably good heart health at all ages.

The Oriental Way to Artery-Washing

For many centuries, Orientals have used large amounts of fish oils. Their traditional folk physicians said that fish oils contained "magic" ingredients that helped wash out their arteries and lubricate their joints to give them the youthfulness of young warriors. What is the "magic" or "secret" ingredient?

Today we know that oils extracted from fatty fishes have *polyunsaturated* ingredients, which are effective in helping to lower the cholesterol level in the blood. The benefit here is that these artery-washing oils remain polyunsaturated because they are never hydrogenated; the lecithin is never removed. The chains of the essential fatty acids remain intact and promote an internal action that helps to break up the cholesterol deposits into tinier particles, then to be distributed throughout the body. As such, the "secret ingredient" of the polyunsaturated factor in fish oils helps to metabolize (break and distribute small cholesterol deposits) the accumulated fats and carry them via the bloodstream to the "ports-of-call" throughout the body. This is a natural "artery-washing" secret long used by the Orientals to help keep their arteries and heart feeling youthfully oiled and lubricated.

The Secret Power of Fish Oils

Fish oils are prime sources of magnesium, a mineral that combines with iodine and promotes a better metabolization of cholesterol. The ocean contains just about all the known minerals, and fish oils are prime sources of such artery-washing minerals. This may well be the secret of the lubricating power of fish oils, and the Orientals swear by this health-building secret.

The Oils That Help Promote Heart Health: The same oils used by the Orientals are available at almost every food store or supermarket as well as most health food stores. Such oils include: olive oil; sesame seed oil; soybean oil; almond oil; peanut oil; walnut oil; corn oil; safflower oil; sunflower oil; wheat germ oil; rice germ oil.

Fish oils used by the Orientals are codfish liver oil, halibut liver oil, whale liver oil as well as oils from tuna or salmon. *Note:* When purchasing oils, use the free-flowing cold-pressed, non-hydrogenated variety sold at most markets and health stores. Read the label. The more natural and non-processed the oil, the more beneficial it should be for your heart and health.

Secret Power of Plant and Seed Oils

Vegetable and seed oils offer an outstanding combination of cholesterol-lowering factors; this was discovered long ago by the Orientals. Modern knowledge tells us that we have these three secrets of the heart rejuvenating benefits of plant and seed oils:

1. A desirable ratio of polyunsaturated to saturated fat.
2. A larger percentage of cholesterol-lowering plant-seed ingredients than any other source.
3. A favorable proportion of all the essential fatty acid components.

In combination, these three benefits unite in plant or seed oils and work to help metabolize the various atoms of carbon, hydrogen and oxygen, linked together in chains that may become thick accumulations of cholesterol. The Oriental dependence upon and faith in plant and seed oils for self-washing has proven its wisdom. Today, the Asiatic people have a much lower incidence of artery-heart distress as compared to the "hard" fat-eating Americans and Europeans. The Orientals have tapped the secrets of their ancestral folk physicians, blended them with modern scientific knowledge of heart-health programs and emerged as youthfully healthy people.

The Yoga Breathing Exercise That Sends Healing Oxygen to the Heart

For the people of India and the surrounding Eurasian nations, yoga is more than just a way of life — it is a way of health. Yoga reportedly offers many healing powers and will help promote better aeration of the heart. For many yoga devotees, a "secret" breathing exercise — known as *shavasan* — is as beneficial to the heart as a supply of oxygen from a tank. The peoples of India, unable to obtain or afford adequate medical help, developed different yoga exercises and also created other folk programs designed to help create natural healing with the use of free and natural methods. One such natural healing program is this *shavasan* — the yoga way to send healing oxygen to the heart with simple breathing exercises.

How Shavasan Acts as a Natural Oxygen Tank

When Middle Eastern folks want to send healing oxygen to the heart, they perform this simple yoga exercise:

Lie flat on your back in a tranquil place. Very slowly, breathe in and breathe out. Concentrate first on the *cooling* effect in your nostrils as you breathe in. Then concentrate on the *warming* effect as you breathe out. Continue this shavasan secret exercise for up to ten minutes during any given day.

Benefits: The secret here is that shavasan helps lower a figurative pressure gauge in the hypothalamas (that part of the brain which influences heart-related body functions, such as blood pressure). This *steady shavasan breathing* appears to lower and then stabilize this figurative pressure gauge. A relaxation of blood pressure enables heart-healing oxygen to go streaming throughout the heart via the rejuvenated blood-stream. The rhythmic shavasan exercises work simultaneously to promote this oxygenation of the heart and to normalize blood pressure. The result is better heart health and body rejuvenation.

Doctors Report on the Heart-Health Benefits of Shavasan[1]

A team of doctors worked with 47 patients in Bombay, India. There were 37 men and 10 women treated for problems of hypertension, kidney malfunction and arteriosclerosis. Needless to say, these patients exhibited varying degrees of heart malfunctioning; yet, when they performed the simple shavasan exercises, their conditions improved and their drug dosages were constantly reduced.

Natural Healing: The majority of the 47 patients showed improvements in their symptoms. Headache, nervousness, irritability and insomnia were relieved in almost all of them. The other symptoms became less marked; in general, the patients experienced a sense of youthful well-being after this all-natural shavasan exercise. It was noted that their conditions improved and that they might soon be considered well — all this as a result of a traditional shavasan exercise, performed under the observation of American physicians.

Yoga Posture Helps Regulate Blood Pressure and Soothe the Heart

The simple prone position (lying flat on the back) while performing rhythmic breathing exercises has a benefit that regulates the blood pressure and soothes the heart. This simple posture helps to lower the systolic and diastolic blood pressure readings, and thereby helps soothe an overworked heart.

Shavasan helps promote a natural form of relaxation through its concentration on good posture. It is soothing to straighten the back and use shavasan breathing to help keep the internal organs in better alignment. Just 30 minutes of this exercise helps cool off those steamed-up tensions that erupt first in the

---

[1]From a speech before the Joint Annual Meeting of the American College of Angiology and International College of Angiology, Las Vegas, Nevada, 1967.

form of high blood pressure and then in oxygen-starved heart distress.

Best Yoga Posture: Lie supine, with your legs at 30 degree angles to your body; your arms should be held comfortably by your sides. Breathe gently and relax your way to better aeration of your heart and bloodstream.

Benefit: In this position, renin activity in the bloodstream is much lower. (Renin is a component of blood associated with kidney-caused high blood pressure.) The shavasan posture enables the renin to remain at a lower level, which helps reduce the incidence of high blood pressure and related heart distress.

Simple? Yes. Effective? Look to the superior health of the many practitioners of yoga and shavasan as your proof that this is another secret from the Orient that deserves practice in the Western world.

Two Secrets of the Heart-Healthy Yogi

Yoga devotees hold that shavasan is a "natural oxygen tank," but that better heart health calls for natural living programs such as:

1. A settled mind in which there is a program of regular relaxation and cleansing of the evil poisons of selfishness, greed and hatred.

2. A more healthful diet, which calls for elimination of salt and spicy condiments. The yogi devotees prefer raw vegetables, abundant cooked soybeans and available fresh fruits. Those who eat animal products prefer very lean or fat-trimmed meats as well as freshly prepared fish.

These two "secrets" are surprisingly similar to the programs offered to patients in the Western world after they have experienced heart attacks. The difference between the Orient and the West is that in the Orient, natural health programs are followed to *prevent* illness; in the West, such programs are usually resorted to *after* an illness occurs. The Oriental folk physicians admonished their followers to align with Nature and fortify health to avoid any such illnesses.

In shavasan, we see that the secret healing power is for the practitioner to drift away from outside influences. He uses his mind in a form of astral projection — to concentrate so deeply upon his health that the breathing ritual enables the body to become totally limp. Here we see the most perfect form of relaxation for someone who fears heart distress. Shavasan offers tranquility to the related blood circulation and heart networks and helps send a stream of life-giving oxygen to this master organ of the body.

The Orientals are known for having the lowest incidence of heart distress in our modern times. Their secrets call for natural living programs based upon traditional folk physicians' secrets — as beneficial today as they were in the past.

IMPORTANT POINTS:

1. Plant or fish oils have been prescribed as "heart-washing" liquids by Oriental folk physicians — and by modern scientists, too.
2. Paul L. changed to the "right kind of Oriental fat" and experienced better heart health, freedom from chest pains and more youthful energy. He now enjoys all the taste of fat with less of the harmful consequences by following Oriental programs.
3. The Orientals recognize that using "right" instead of "wrong" fats maintains a heart-healthy yin-yang balance.
4. The Orientals use fish oils as a "secret" way to wash their arteries and promote youthful health for the heart.
5. Plant and seed oils offer "secret" cholesterol-washing benefits enjoyed by the healthy Orientals.
6. Shavasan is a yoga breathing exercise that takes just 30 minutes a day, yet reportedly helps promote natural oxygenation in the heart, soothing tranquilization, better sleeping and more youthful vitality.

14

The Magic Healing Power of
Tibetan Herbs

Forbidden Tibet has long held the secrets of perpetual youth and health, guarded jealously by a select few monks who inscribed treasured potions and remedies that reportedly could bring about rejuvenation of the mind and body. These secrets were painstakingly recorded in holy scrolls, which were kept guarded in the mysterious Tibetan temples. It took hundreds of centuries for the secrets to make their way through the treacherous mountain reaches, by way of voyagers and explorers, down to the Orient, where they were found to possess magic healing powers.

Youthful Healing from a Divine Source

Folk legend tells us that the ancient Tibetan lamas taught that youthful healing and the secret of eternal life could come solely from a divine source. These high priests further taught that the body was inviolate and could not be desecrated by instruments. They expounded the revelation that because the body was a creation of divine sources, youthful healing would come from other creations of the great deities of the heavens. Herbs were considered life-giving medicines from celestial gardeners, made available for believers who sought eternal youth and health. The Tibetan monks prepared many scrolls

174

describing such youthful healing herbs, and they recorded many case histories of Tibetans who lived for several hundred years in youthful good health, through the judicious use of such secret herbs. Considering that modern scientists have corroborated the vigorous good health of these Tibetans, it is reasonable to believe that there is a magic healing power in their herbs.

Eternal Youth Cult Created
by Herb-Worshipping Tibetans

Because the Tibetan herbs did, indeed, help promote magic healing, the Tibetan leaders formed a cult devoted to the use of these secret life-giving medicines from the celestial deities.

The followers jealously guarded their secrets of youth. Locked high in the unapproachable mountain peaks of the Himalayas, within the crevices and hollowed-out secret cities near Mt. Everest, close to 30,000 feet up toward the heavens, the youth cult worshipped the herbs that their lamas promised would give them eternal life. They developed the Mahayana Buddhism cult which was marked by tantric and shamanistic rituals and a dominant hierarchical monasticism. Locked within the monasteries of the lamas, the secret herbs were described, grown and used as part of the worship of the eternal youth cult.

The Lamaist monks described their youth-giving herbs in the tantric scriptures, enshrouded in mysticism and magic and embodying the worship of Shakti, a deity who was said to hold the secret of eternal vitality and perpetual life. From legends and factual reports that drifted down the impassable peaks of the Himalayan mountains, many learned that the Tibetans did have the secret of perpetual youth and health. The Tibetans sought to keep their secrets for themselves, fearing that outsiders would invade their lands and desecrate their holy shrines. But Oriental spies sent to Tibet by surrounding rulerships were able to bring back some of the coveted herbs and stories of the amazing centuries-old cultists from this magic land. Slowly, the secrets sifted out and the same herbs could be grown in other Oriental countries to offer hope for perpetual youth and health.

Early Oriental Writings
About Tibetan Youth Herbs

Back in the fog of antiquity, some 5,000 years ago, Emperor Shen Nung, in his *Pen-ts'ao* (a compendium of natural remedies), described the magic Tibetan herbs and how the taking of them could alleviate illnesses and extend life. Several centuries afterwards, Emperor Huang Ti, in his celebrated *Nei Ching,* told of sending emissaries to Tibet, disguised as pilgrims and seekers of divine truth. The emissaries had been schooled in the Tibetan dialect and masqueraded as lamas from a distant and unapproachable settlement in the Himalayas. Thus, they gained entrance into the holy lamasery of the three-century old Imperial Lama, and were given a set of herbal secrets of perpetual youth. These emissaries took handfuls of herbs from the sacred gardens surrounding the lamasery and returned to Emperor Huang Ti with their precious booty. The herbs were described in the *Nei Ching,* and it is further reported they produced miracle healing powers and extended the lives of many who used them regularly.

Much later, about 450 A.D., a court-appointed physician and alchemist, T'ao Hung-ching, prepared a handbook describing many Tibetan and Oriental herbs and extolled their virtues and magical powers of life and health. He said that judicious use of such Tibetan herbs could offer hope for eternal youth. The fact that those who took such Tibetan herbs did experience healthful recovery (but not, of course, eternal life) did offer a promise for better living with these magical substances. Many Oriental scholars felt that the secrets of the Tibetan lamas were still hidden and that the *combination* of herbs (the formulae still hidden in the Tibetan lamasery) could offer eternal life. This led to various experiments of herbal combinations that were recorded in more Oriental scrolls, and kept even until this day.

The most recent work was the *Pen-ts'ao Kang-mu* (Pharmacopoeia) prepared by Li Shih-chen, a respected physician who lived towards the end of the 16th century (he is revered in modern China as a scholar and healer). Li Shih-chen listed a number of Tibetan herbs and said that they could promote youthful health. He promised eternal life as suggested by the Tibetan monks, but said that the secret was in a proper *com-*

bination of such herbs in a proper amount. This secret is yet to be discovered, but it does offer hope for lasting youth, as promised by the centuries-old but youthfully healthy Tibetan monks.

The Tibetan Herb That is Worshipped as the "Elixir of Life"

Fo-ti-Tieng (botanically known as *Hydrocotyle asiatica minor*) is a Tibetan herb that has long been worshipped as the "elixir of life." As living proof, past and present scientists have told of the long life enjoyed by the Oriental herbalist, Li Chung Yun.

It is said that Professor Li Chung Yun offered documents to show that he was born in 1677. He died in 1933 — *enjoying a life span of 256 years!!* These documents reportedly showed that he had survived 23 wives and was living happily with his 24th wife at the time of his passing. The Chinese Government sent the respected dean of the Chang-Tu University, Professor Wu Chung Chich, to research facts offered by the long-living Li Chung Yun. In a short time, Professor Wu Shung Chich corroborated all that the centuries-old Oriental had said — that he was, indeed, well over 250 years of age! Furthermore, he said that the secret of living a long and youthful life was in the Tibetan herb, Fo-ti-Tieng.

As a botanist, Li Chung Yun cultivated many herbs in his private garden, but specialized in Fo-ti-Tieng. He would take it in the form of a tea, which he would drink as often as five times daily. Whenever he felt "weak," he would bolster his youthful vitality with this Tibetan herb, which had already become known to the Orientals as the "elixir of life."

More Health Secrets of the 256 Year-Young Man

A professor at Minkuo University, near Peking, reported that this 256-year-young man stood straight and strong, had his own teeth and a full head of healthy hair. Li Chung Yun said that he had learned other secrets from Tibetan travelers, namely, to remain calm and peaceful, to walk upright and to sleep like a babe. He said that the Tibetan monks suggested taking Fo-ti-Tieng daily, along with the ginseng root. Most important, they advised youth-seekers to *eat food that is grown above the ground* (the ginseng root being the only exception).

This suggests adherence to a vegetarian program — one that reportedly gave Li Chung Yun two-and-a-half centuries of youthful health. His demise occurred when Oriental scholars and botanists came to his herbal garden and dug up the precious "elixir of life," depriving him of his source of health. Denied Fo-ti-Tieng, he succumbed.

Youth Substances in the Tibetan Herb. The leaves and the seeds of the herb are said to possess an alkaloid, which promotes a revitalizing effect in the cellular networks and tissue enclosures of the brain and nervous system. A "missing substance" rarely found in other foods appears to be present in Fo-ti-Tieng and helps to stimulate the ductless glands, enabling them to send forth a steady supply of hormones (rivers of youth) throughout the body. This is said to help nourish all body organs, and to bring about a rejuvenating effect.

Health Benefits of the Tibetan Herb. The tonifying ingredients work within the metabolic system to help improve the enzyme flow (needed for digestive juices and subsequent assimilation of nutrients), help regulate the delicate metabolic process and establish the coveted yin-yang balance of youthful health. Ingredients in Fo-ti-Tieng appear to enter into most of the body processes and can rightfully be considered the "elixir of life," according to the long-living Tibetans and their latest living proof, the 256-year-young Li Chung Yun.

The Secret Tibetan Herb That Renews the Cells and Tissues

Modern science explains that the cells and tissues of the human body do not age. Every single moment, millions of cells and tissues become deficient in their biologic activity. They are given off through wastes and the body then creates new cells and tissues to replace those that have died. A modern fact is that *every two years, nearly 92% of the body cells and tissues are regenerated.* Nature works to provide youthful new cells but *not* aged cells. Nature derives her working materials from foods that are ingested. When you give Nature all the vital ingredients needed, it is possible for this cellular rejuvenation process to continue indefinitely.

Although the Tibetans may have lacked our modern microscopic and chemical apparatus, they did have divine wisdom and knew that cellular-tissue rejuvenation could be continued "forever" with the proper ingredients.

They learned that one herb reportedly possessed this treasure of divine ingredients and offered hope for perpetual youth through cellular-tissue rejuvenation. The herb came to be known as *Gotu Kola*. Forbidden Tibetan scrolls described Gotu Kola as an "eternal life" plant and said that it could be recognized as a small plant that kept close to the soil; it had pale-green, fan-shaped leaves.

The taste of Gotu Kola is somewhat strong, but when eaten together with a whole-grain food, it is most flavorful. Orientals believe that this herb holds the Tibetan promise of eternal life, and they eat it just as they would a youth elixir or aphrodisiac.

The Gotu Kola Renews Cells and Tissues and Energizes Body Functions

Special substances and oils found within the leaves of the Gotu Kola reportedly help create cellular rejuvenation. These substances offer the metabolic processes and the needed working materials from which new cells are made. This plant also rejuvenates the cells and tissues of the brain and the various body organs, and it is sent into the bloodstream, where it helps send essential ingredients to other parts of the body. This creates a feeling of internal rejuvenation through energizing and re-activating sluggish processes. These were the revitalizations experienced by Tibetans, hence their promise, "Two leaves a day will keep old age away." Many Tibetan lamas would use the leaves daily as a means of stimulating their psychic powers and developing their occult facilities. Today, we interpret these functions as "brain regeneration."

Live Beyond the Century Mark. For many centuries, Gotu Kola has been growing throughout India, where travelers planted it as soon as they descended the steep Himalayas of forbidden

Tibet. The plant now flourishes throughout India and Ceylon. Natives say that it helps improve the youth of the brain, gives them strength and helps them live beyond the century mark. Many Indian and Ceylonese do live past the age of 100 and they attribute this to their regular use of this Tibetan herb.

Cellular Rejuvenation is a Secret of Eternal Youth. Modern science knows that perpetual youth may be possible if the process of cellular rejuvenation is continued indefinitely, and the Tibetan lamas held that the secret of eternal youth was in the Gotu Kola. This magic herb promotes an indefinite cellular rejuvenation reaction that may well be the most sacred secret of the holy Lamas, who lived for hundreds of years in a state of lasting youth!

Herb Secrets from the Monasteries of Tibet

Voyagers, explorers and caravan masters who travelled throughout the Orient and ventured in or near Tibet were able to wrest some herb secrets from bribe-greedy gardeners and less-devout natives. Slowly, herb secrets were made known. Botanists were able to identify these herbs and found that they could flourish in most soils throughout Europe and (later) America.

A group of Tibetan youth-giving herbs, which are now available at most herbal pharmacies and health food shoppes, is made up of the following:

Acacia. Also known as gum arabic and gum acacia, this herb helps to relax and renew the cells and tissues and promote a healthful astringent to the surface of the skin.

Agar. An Oriental algae that is harvested in the late summer, then sun-dried, boiled and turned into a mucilaginous liquid, its jelly-like form is good in cooked dishes. It reportedly helps smooth and wash debris from the internal organs, promoting a sparkling clean feeling from the inside.

Aloes. This is said to help cleanse the colon, scrub away infectious wastes and age-causing deterioration (mucous wastes), and expel "evil spirits" from the intestinal canal. Today, such "evil spirits" are identified as pinworms.

Anise. This Tibetan herb features many oil-filled globules; when inhaled, these help to dispel tiredness and promote energy and vitality. When the anise herb is used as a flavoring agent, it has a regenerating benefit to the internal viscera.

Asafetida. Also known as gum asafetida, this herb has a powdered gum resin that is said to help regenerate the brain and the cerebro-nervous system. It also helps to tone up sluggish organs to create a feeling of youthful vitality.

How Ella L. Uses Asafetida as a Mind Tonic: Ella L. works long hours as a researcher, and she feels that she needs something to perk up her mind. She obtains asafetida in powdered form, dissolves one half teaspoon in two cups of boiled water and, when cooled, she sips several tablespoons while working. She finds that this gives her a feeling of mental alertness. Ingredients in this Tibetan herb help give her a relaxed sensation of warmth, yet there is no increase in temperature. She finds that this simple Tibetan secret offers her a "mind tonic" that enables her to work long hours.

Balm. Also called sweet balm, garden balm and lemon balm, this locally available Tibetan herb can be made into a refreshing tea. Lamasery monks reported that it helped rejuvenate the viscera such as the kidneys, spleen, bladder and liver.

Balm of Gilead. Tibetans valued this herb for its ability to help soothe distress in the stomach, lungs, kidneys and chest. Scholars reported that when blended with an ointment (such as our modern vaseline) and rubbed on the skin, it helped bring about healing of blemishes, helped erase wrinkles and promoted a youthful skin-glow.

Benne. In modern language, this is known as sesame. The Tibetans used the seeds and leaves in hot water for a tea, to help rejuvenate the respiratory tract — notably the lungs and bronchial tubes. They believed that good breathing was symbolic of perpetual youth, and they said that this herb helped promote youthful breathing.

Burdock. Tibetans praised the youth-building powers of this herb. In modern terms, it helps stimulate the flow of enzymes in the digestive tract. The key to longevity is often traced to healthy enzymatic, digestive-assimilative powers and burdock is believed to help rejuvenate the digestive system and spark the flow of much-needed enzyme juices.

Cinnamon. The powdered cinnamon bark is said to promote an astringent benefit to enable cellular tissues to contract and expel wastes. It is this self-cleansing action which caused cinnamon to be a much-revered herb in the Tibetan monasteries.

Cloves. Aromatic oils of cloves contain ingredients that help stabilize blood circulation and regulate body temperature. Cloves are said to promote enzymatic flow and thereby boost youthful digestive functioning. So-called arthritic-like muscular cramps are often relieved when the oil of cloves is applied as a poultice near an affected region. Tibetans prized the oil of cloves for its pain-easing powers.

Ergot. This reportedly helps rejuvenate the glands of the body. In particular, ergot is said to help soothe problems of an enlarged prostate gland in the male. Ingredients in ergot reportedly act as an aphrodisiac through glandular rejuvenation. Tibetan monks were forbidden the use of ergot because of a vow of celibacy. But they gave this aphrodisiac to worshippers who were impotent or childless and they reported rejuvenation among the devout believers.

Horehound. The dried leaves and flowering tops of this plant reportedly have the ability to help slough off age-causing debris particles from tissue membranes throughout the body. Mix the juice of this herb with honey to help promote healing of ulcerated sores and blemishes.

Hyssop. Hyssop leaves are said to contain oils that act as general cleansers and purifiers throughout the body. In the Bible (John 19:28, 29,) hyssop is referred to as a holy herb. Traditionally, Tibetan lamas would offer hyssop to their deities during sacred and secret services.

Juniper Berry. This reportedly acts as a stimulant to sluggish body functions. In particular, it helps regulate the yin-yang balance of liquid in the body to help ease problems of accumulations of fluids. Tibetan monks also called this herb the "fruit of passion" because it was known to act as an aphrodisiac in men and women.

Sarsaparilla. When troubled by pains in the head or joints of the body, sarsaparilla is reported to be soothing and healing. It was held in high esteem by Tibetan monks because it purified the blood, counteracted debilitating infections, stimulated the glands and helped nullify the harmful effects of toxic wastes.

Tansy. This herb is said to promote uterine rejuvenation in the female. Also, it reportedly helps soothe nervous unrest and promotes a general tranquility of the spirits.

Wormwood. The Tibetans prized this herb because it had a strange ingredient (identified as absinthe, or an aphrodisiac), which was said to promote romanticism in men or women. It was denied use by the celibate Tibetan monks, but it was given to those devout followers who displayed symptoms of impotence or frigidity.

How to Purchase Herbs

Look in the yellow pages of your local telephone directory for businesses in your region. If you reside in a very small town, consult the directory of the nearest large city in your area. Look under these classifications: *Botanicals, Health Food Stores, Herbs, Oils, Perfumes (raw materials), Sachets, Spices.*

Also: Look under *Pharmacy* and ask where such herbs are available if the pharmacy does not have them.

For youthful health tap the secrets of the Tibetans, who trusted Nature because they knew that youth and health came from divine sources.

SUMMARY:

1. The Tibetan monks probed the secrets of eternal life, reportedly enjoyed centuries of youthful life and believed that magic herbs provided the source of forever-young health.
2. An eternal youth cult created by herb-worshipping Tibetans held the secret of perpetual life.
3. The Fo-ti-Tieng herb, available in most modern herb stores, reportedly enabled a man to live to be 256 years of age. The Tibetans prized this secret herb as an "elixir of life."

4. The Gotu Kola herb, described in secret and forbidden Tibetan scrolls, helps to rejuvenate the cells and tissues and prompt a form of self-renewal that holds the key to eternal life.

5. Tibetan herbs are cultivated locally and made available for your use. Ella L. uses asafetida as a natural mind tonic. Other described herbs offer Tibetan-reported secrets of magic rejuvenation and perpetual life.

15

Oriental Reflexology: The Natural Way to Help Heal Muscular Aches and Pains

Oriental reflexology is a once-secret method of helping to loosen up knotted muscles and promote free-flowing circulation. The Orientals understood that youthful suppleness, muscular agility and limb flexibility could be enjoyed when a series of simple, all-natural remedial massage practices were applied to the body. It was their "secret" of helping to relieve such distress symptoms as stiff muscles and aching limbs.

Today, we recognize these muscular pains as arthritic-like symptoms, but to the ancient Oriental, they were the reactions of a maladjusted *yin-yang* balance. It was Oriental reflexology that helped restore this balance and enable the body to recover from muscular soreness and stiffness.

How Reflexology Soothes Muscles, Relaxes the Body, Stimulates Circulation and Induces Sleep

Wise Oriental physicians reported that man's first medical tool was *his own hand.* Whenever a man was hurt, seized with a pain, he instinctively placed his hand to the aching spot to offer protection, or to rub, knead or massage. These instinctive reflex motions were recorded thousands of years ago in Oriental

185

medical scrolls. The traditionally wise Oriental physicians explained that if this instinctive "hand upon the pain" could help soothe, relax, stimulate and induce a feeling of contentment, then this "medical tool" could be used for the entire body to induce youthful health. From this simple observation, the Oriental healing secret of reflexology was born to provide merciful healing of aches and pains for many privileged royalists.

Secrets Described in Hidden Scrolls

During the Han period in China (206-220 A.D.), royal physicians described the methods of reflexology for healing muscular aches and pains in such private and secret scrolls as *The Yellow Emperor's Classic of Internal Medicine, Book of Medicaments of Shen-nung, Short Version of the Golden Shrine* and the *Book of the Pulse.*

At this time in Oriental history, the patrician aristocracy held the power in the villages. The royalists formed alliances with Buddhist leaders of India and soon exchanged healing secrets; however, knowledge of reflexology was restricted to a chosen few. Caravaners often brought along an Oriental physician who would treat royalists in distant lands, relieving their arthritic-like muscular distress and restoring them to such youthful health that trade flourished and lucrative import-export agreements were offered as "rewards" for such healing.

During the 4th century A.D., the book *Pao P'u-tzu* was made available to a few royalists. This work described many of the methods of natural healing that we know today as Oriental reflexology. The subsequent *Thousand Ducat Prescriptions* was prepared during the T'ang Dynasty, from 618 to 907 A.D. Crude methods of printing had begun to be used during this period, but more important, this dynasty saw the establishment of the first school of medicine and the beginnings of a medical library to serve the students and physicians. Since this occurred at the time when printing was being developed, it meant that many of the once-secret Oriental medical books could now be printed for the students of the university. This was done at the urging of many Oriental physicians who sought to bring healing to the common people. In particular, Ko Hung (in the 4th century), T'ao Hung-ching (in the 5th century) and the brilliant Sun Szumiao (581-682 A.D.) pleaded for dissemination of methods of reflexology, among other natural healing programs, to help bring youthful health to so many sufferers.

Thus was born the Oriental method of healing that we know today as reflexology. It was taught as a subject in many Oriental medical schools, and became more popular during the Ming dynasty (1368-1644) as a method of helping to restore youthful flexibility to aching limbs.

Benefit of Oriental Reflexology

Oriental textbooks explained that reflexology, known as *An-mo* or *T'ui-na,* was completely drugless and required no medication or special instruments. It needed only one's own (or an aid's) healing hands. Self-massage or finger-pressure stimulation, which is the basis of reflexology, seeks to move sluggish fatty tissue to stimulate the receptors in the skin. This encourages a youthful blood flow and, according to reflexology teachers, helps to balance the *yin-yang* stress ratio. Reflexology benefits by alerting sluggish muscular metabolism, firming up weakened muscles and soothing cramps.

The *An-mo* method of reflexology works to *press* and *rub* the aching region. This helps tone the body.

The *T'ui-na* method of reflexology works to *thrust* and *roll* the aching region. This helps relax and soothe the body.

The 8 Secret Reflexology Motions
That Help Melt Aches and Pains

Here are 8 reflexology motions that reportedly will help promote remedial healing of aches and pains. The Oriental physicians suggested that the individual locate his distress spot, then apply the following do-it-yourself healing motions:

1. Thrusting (T'ui). Use the thumb or the ball of your thumb.

(a) *Perpendicular Thrusting (P'ing-t'ui).* Place your thumb, or the ball of your thumb, upon the sore spot and make a continuous gentle pressure movement in a vertical direction. *Benefit:* This helps soothe aches of the chest, lumbar region, stomach, arms and legs.

(b) *Lateral Thrusting (Ts'e-t'ui).* Place your thumb or the ball of your thumb upon the sore spot and make a continuous gentle pressure movement but in a horizontal-lateral direction. *Benefit:* This helps increase sluggish blood circulation in the head and neck.

(c) *Plane Thrusting (Pao-t'ui).* Place your thumb, or the ball of your thumb, upon the sore spot and move backwards and forwards in a continuous gentle pressure movement *Benefit:* This helps loosen up tight knots in the region of the chest and legs.

(d) *Semi-Circular Thrusting (Ch-an-ta).* Use the edge of your thumb upon the sore spot. Use quick motions in a semi-circular gentle pressure movement. *Benefit:* This helps soothe and relax sore spots on the rib region of the chest and the stomach.

2. Grasping (Na). This secret method calls for using a gentle shaking or vibrating motion. Gradually, you firm up the grasp. It helps tone up aching muscles and loosen up knotted or gnarled joints. Oriental scholars presented these four variations of grasping:

(a) *Muscle Rolling (Chan-chuan-fa).* With your fingertips, gently grasp individual muscle cords. Roll backwards; roll forwards; use a linear or circular motion. For painful extremities, roll the grasped muscle cords between the palms of your hands; for example, a painful calf muscle may thus be invigorated and soothed by muscle rolling between your palms.

(b) *Shrinking (Chin-so-na).* Gently grasp the muscles and skin on your neck and shoulders into folds. Repeat as often as desired.

(c) *Shaking (Yao-fa).* With your fingertips, gently grasp individual muscle cords. Shake vigorously backwards and forwards to help loosen up congestion. This is especially soothing to the painful knots of the nape of the neck and the region of the sacrum.

(d) *Vibrating (Tou-fa).* Press your fingertips on the skin above the aching region. Move your fingertips very gently in a back-and-forth rhythm. This is very beneficial to aching limbs.

3. Pressing (An). Use your entire palm for maximum healing benefits. If the region is too painful, use fingertips and gradually increase to the entire palm as healing is experienced. Here are the methods:

(a) *Finger Pressing (Chih-an).* Use gentle to gradually stronger pressure with up to five fingertips on the aching region. Orientalists prescribed this for the head, neck, lumbar regions and legs.

(b) *Palm Pressing (Ch'ang-an).* Gently press your entire palm upon the aching region and rub very soothingly. This is especially beneficial for aches in the region of the stomach.

(c) *Thumb Tip Pressing (Tien-an).* Gentle pressing upon the aching portion with the thumb tip is said to help free congestion in the region.

4. Rubbing (Mo-fa). Use the ball of your thumb, your palm or your fingers upon the aching region. Rub with quick motions Be gentle. Increase rubbing pressures as you experience relief.

5. Back of the Hand Rolling (Kun-fa). Make a clenched fist. Use the back of the fist in a gentle rocking pressure motion over the aching region. Oriental folk healers stressed gentleness and a gradual increase in pressure as healing and strengthening were experienced.

6. Pinching (Nieh-fa). Use your thumb and index finger. Seize the skin and muscle segments and use your thumb and index fingers as "pincers" to press, then release, then press again. *Tip:* Do this in the direction of the muscle fiber. This helps promote gentle healing and stimulates sluggishness and congestion.

7. Palm Rubbing (Ch'a-fa). Seize the affected region such as the legs (ankle, calf muscles, knee, thigh) or any other accessible body part. Rub between your palms, using gentle-to-vigorous pressure. This helps liberate sluggish congestion of these aching regions.

8. Tapping (P'o-fa). Use your palm, the back of your hand, your fist or even the side of your hand. Gently "tap" the stiff portion. Keep up a steady rhythm and increase the force of the tapping as you experience relief from aching.

Secret Benefits of
Do-It-Yourself Oriental Reflexology

The gentle form of reflexology offers a tonifying benefit; the more vigorous form of reflexology offers a sedating benefit. The Chinese work, *Synopsis of the Technique of Remedial Massage,* published in 1889, recommends Oriental reflexology because of its healing benefits. These Oriental scholars believe that reflexology works on the "gate control" theory.

According to this theory, sensations traveling along peripheral nerve fibers must pass through a figurative gate in the spinal cord before they are transmitted upward to the brain. Pain is transmitted along relatively thin fibers and tends to keep the gate open. But impulses such as those involving vibratory sensation and position sense travel over a larger type of fiber and override the pain sensation at the spinal cord.

Hand pressure reflexology upon these fibers helps produce a vibratory stimulus that closes the gate and blocks the transmission of pain to the brain.

Secret: The "gate control secret" of pain holds that specific nerve cells in the spinal cord can either inhibit or intensify the flow of pain impulses to the brain. Reflexology benefits by preventing pain in two ways: (1) By blocking the transmission of pain sensations from peripheral nerves to the spinal cord and thus to the brain. (2) By shutting down the pain reception center in the brain itself. *Benefit:* Since various nerve "circuits" control the organs, reflexology helps relieve pain even when pressure is exerted upon regions other than the affected parts. This helps restore the balance of Yin and Yang and promote restoration of health and a natural way to relieve muscular aches and pains, according to the Orientals. In brief, restore the flow of energy to the afflicted region and youthful vitality may well be the reward.

How Gerald V. Uses Six-Minute Reflexology
to Relieve Headaches and Refresh Tired Eyes

Schoolteacher Gerald V. uses his eyes to the straining extreme. In addition to daily classwork, he must also use his eyes in the evenings and many weekends for correcting homework and also for preparing examinations as well as for grading them.

Aspirin Allergy Leads to Discovery of Oriental Headache-Eye Remedy. Gerald V. tried many medicinal headache remedies and different types of aspirin. Almost always, he had adverse reactions and side effects. He thought he might have to suffer recurring headaches and eye distress, until he complained to a fellow schoolteacher who had just returned from a sabbatical in the Orient. The friend told of a traditional Oriental folk remedy for headaches that also refreshed tired eyes. He said that it had been used for thousands of years and that it was currently in use, since modern patent medicines are either unknown or unavailable in the Orient. Gerald V. tried this simple and effective Oriental remedy.

Relax-Refresh With K'an-kung Stimulation (T'ui K'an-kung-fa). Place the balls of both thumbs on the "points" found just above your eyebrows. (These are called the *K'an-kung* points.) Massage these points very gently. Then push outwardly — that is, your right thumb pushes the *K'an-kung* or above-eyebrow region toward the right. Your left thumb pushes the *K'an-kung* or above-eyebrow region toward the left. Continue for up to ten minutes. Oriental healers suggested following this simple, relaxing reflexological remedy at least twice daily. It was said to relieve the headaches and eyestrain of the Oriental scholars who had to squint and strain to write the complicated brush strokes of Chinese and Japanese characters. It was a remedy born out of necessity.

How Gerald Achieved Healing Relief from Headaches. Gerald V. was unable to take aspirins, because of their side effects; so he used this all-natural reflexological method. He discovered at first that it would ease headaches and relieve eyestrain; later, he found a feeling of delightful refreshment as head pains subsided and his eyesight became clearer and better. Now, Gerald V. enjoys freedom from recurring headaches, thanks to this reflexological secret from the past.

How Peggy J. Relieves Stiff Wrists With a Reflexology Secret from India

Close to 2,000 years ago, Manu, the Hindu law-giver, prepared a set of rules for long life and youthful health. This Hindu saint heard of reflexology and prepared several "secrets" to be used by those who wanted to tap the wellsprings of perpetual youth.

One such "secret" called for simple remedial motions that were said to help "close the gate" to the pathway of pain. Reportedly, it was said to help loosen up stiff limbs.

Bookkeeper Peggy Taps Secret of Sacred Manu. As a bookkeeper, Peggy J. had to use her fingers almost all day long. If she was not writing numbers in long columns, she was using a typewriter or adding machine. She complained of stiff fingers and thought she was developing symptoms of arthritis. Nothing seemed to help in the way of diathermy or commercial medicines. Her wrists and elbows began to feel so stiff that it was agonizing to bend her fingers to grip a pencil. Warning spasms and tightening made her forearm muscles constrict, and she noticed that her fingers were becoming swollen and gnarled. Her work suffered; she had to do something. While attending a local lecture, she noted a demonstration of Eastern and Oriental healing methods. She noted one such remedy that the lecturer said had been created by the divine Manu as part of the health secrets of India, given to his devoted followers. Peggy J. was told to follow this simple reflexological exercise at least three times a day, for just five minutes at a time.

Simple, Yet Effective Wrist-Limbering Reflexology. Hold your right wrist with your left hand. Using your right thumb and fingers, knead each finger separately beginning from tip to knuckles. Press firmly. Now hold the fingers of your right hand with your left hand. Circle your wrist with your right hand. Let your fingers rest on the underside of your forearm. Stroke gently and then firmly up to your elbow or "funny bone."

Slowly, fingertip-knead your forearm muscles, using a series of circles. Slowly, move each circle an inch or two closer to your elbow.

Next, bend your elbow and make certain your muscles are relaxed. Stroke your upper arm muscles up to your shoulders. To further benefit, rotate your arm a few times to help liberate your shoulder joint. Continue stroking your biceps.

How long should these exercises last? The Manu suggests no more than two minutes for each arm, or approximately five minutes for both arms. Simple, yet reportedly effective.

Peggy Experiences a Surge of Youthful Flexibility in Her Wrists and Arms. It took up to four days of this regular program until Peggy J. felt a surge of youthfulness flowing through her arms, from her shoulders right down to her fingertips. Now she could hold a pencil, grip any object, let her fingers dance in rhythm over the keys of an adding machine or typewriter. Melted were the painful spasms. Gone were the agonizing aches that shot through her arms whenever she held onto a pencil for a long time. Peggy J. thanked the Hindu lawgiver, Manu, for helping her with this reflexology remedy that was considered sacred for its ability to heal!

Secret of Healing in the Hands. The Oriental felt that the secret of healing was in the palm and fingers of the hand. One ancient Oriental school maintained that the hand was a living replica of the mystical *yin and yang* and could thus induce youthful healing. Massage, finger-pressure acupuncture as well as remedial reflexology using the hands could help produce healing in mysterious, yet effective ways.

The Eight-Step Way to "Forever-Young" Arms and Legs

The Taoists and Buddhists of the Orient devised reflexological motions that reportedly would help promote "forever young" arms and legs. The Buddhists felt that the body must remain as young as possible in order to remain within the grace of the Supreme Deities. In the 6th Century A.D., a Buddhist monk of Indian origin, Bodhidharma, prepared a set of eight steps that were reportedly effective in loosening up tight arms and legs and helping to keep the body supple, flexible and free from the infirmities of age. This abbot, Bodhidharma, held secret classes for the monks in the Shaolin monastery in the province of Honan. His chosen monks reportedly became so supercharged with youthful energy, they were able to battle younger men in the "art of fisticuffs" or *Ch'uan-shu,* and win with accolades. Others marveled at the youthful flexibility and vigor of the older monks and pried loose the secret eight-step program that helped invigorate and rejuvenate the arms and legs.

Note: The monks performed these eight easy steps upon awakening in the morning, before breakfast. Here is the once-secret, eight-step program devised by the divine Buddhist monk, Bodhidharma:

1. Instant Reflexology. Press your right palm against your right temple. Press hard while you endeavor to lower your head to your right shoulder. Continue up to the count of 10. Then do the same with your left palm to your left temple for another count up to 10.

2. Finger-Limbering. Interlace fingers of both hands with palms forward (a traditional Oriental practice). Press palms against your forehead. Now press your forehead forward while your interlaced fingers resist. Continue up to the count of 10.

3. Chest-Limbering. Move interlaced hands to your chest, and now try to pull your fingers apart. Resist your own efforts and press against your chest while doing so. Continue up to the count of 10.

4. Arm-Loosening. Unlock your fingers. Now press palms together. Gently but firmly keep pushing one palm against the other, until you feel a rhythmic pressure flowing through your forearms and elbows. Continue up to the count of 10.

5. Body Invigorator. Both arms should be stretched by your sides. Open and close your fists. Tight . . . tighter . . . tightest . . . Now make a fan of your fingers; raise your arms all the way up, as if you wanted to touch the ceiling. Now move back and touch the wall behind you, without turning around. Drop your arms. Repeat up to the count of 5.

6. Leg and Toe Loosener. Wiggle your toes very vigorously. Turn your soles toward one another. Swing your legs apart in a wide V arc. Close this V arc. Repeat several times. Continue for 5 minutes.

7. Head-Neck Relaxer. Interlace fingers behind the nape of your neck. Now, keep your knees stiff. Lift your right leg until it is comfortably vertical. Hold for the count of 5. Repeat with your left leg. Hold for the count of 5. *Next:* With both heels together as you stand flat on the floor, and your interlaced clasped fingers behind the nape of your neck, try to raise up on your heels, then raise up on your toes. Alternate to the count of 10 for each one.

8. All-Purpose Rejuvenator. Take a deep breath. Breathe out. Repeat for a few moments. Now, bend your knees. Raise your trunk. Visualize yourself pedaling a bicycle. Repeat up to the count of 10.

Benefits of the Buddhist 8-Step Program
for "Forever-Young" Arms and Legs

The ancient Buddhist medical scrolls promised that those who faithfully took care of their bodies would benefit from a feeling of rest and relaxation. The preceding reflexological motions were said to: soothe minor aches and pains; ease simple nervous tension; melt nervous fatique; help boost circulation; relax discomfort; soothe nervous fatique; help awaken sluggish circulation; relieve muscular spasms; create a balm-like relaxation of the muscles and help to promote restful, natural and drug-free sleep. These were the healthful benefits promised to those who followed the all-natural 8-step way to "forever-young" Arms and Legs. They reportedly helped restore youthful flexibility to many who adhered to the principles of treating the *cause* first and the *symptom* second as a means of building youthful health.

The Orientals have always been (and still are) remarkably agile in body and mind; they enjoy free-moving arms and legs. In many parts of the Orient, problems of arthritis or rheumatism are unknown. This freedom from the so-called afflictions of civilization is their reward for placing faith in the natural healing processes of the body, as taught to them by many Oriental physicians and healers. Reflexology is the Oriental way to free oneself from arthritic-like muscular aches and pains. It may well be one of the most important secrets revealed to the Western world in the quest for youthful flexibility of arms and legs.

IMPORTANT POINTS TO REMEMBER:

1. Oriental reflexology is an ancient and secret method of helping to loosen up "knotted" or arthritic-like painful arms and legs. It is all-natural and drugless.
2. To help melt aches and pains, follow the eight reflexology motions right in your own home. It only takes moments, but it offers hope for healing.
3. Gerald V. relieves headaches and refreshes tired eyes with a six-minute reflexology program.
4. Peggy J. relieves stiff "arthritic-like" wrists and fingers with a reflexology secret from India.

5. The Buddhist monk, Bodhidharma, in the 6th Century A.D., discovered eight steps to "forever-young" arms and legs. About ten minutes in the morning and you will help rejuvenate your body and mind and enjoy youthful limbs and freedom from muscular spasms and aches.

16

How to Stay Younger Longer With Prana – The Hindu Secret of "Youth Breath"

In the 6th Century B.C., Oriental healers inscribed the secret of "youth breath" on a set of 12 jade stones. These healers recognized the therapeutic and rejuvenating benefit of properly performed breathing, which came to be known as *Prana*. The Oriental healers suggested these secrets for corrective breathing, which reportedly would help to infuse the body and mind with feelings of perpetual youth:

"This is how breathing must be done: the breath is retained and collected. When it has collected, it expands. When it expands, it goes downwards. When it goes downwards, it becomes quiet. When it has become quiet, it grows firm. When it is firm, it begins to germinate. When it has germinated, it grows. When it has grown, it must be pressed back. When it has been pressed back, it reaches the crown of the head. At the top it presses against the crown of the head, down below it presses downwards. Whosoever follows this principle, lives; whosoever does the contrary, dies."[1]

The Oriental healers prescribed rhythmic breathing, which came to be known as *Prana*, as a means of offering "immortal-

[1]Wilhelm Helmut, *A Chou Inscription on the Technique of Breathing*, quoted by Joseph Needham in "Science and Civilization in China" Vol. II, p. 143. (Cambridge University Press, Cambridge, Mass., 1956)

ity" and youthful health. These same "youth breaths" were
part of the secret teachings of Taoism and Buddhism and,
later, the Hindu religion. As early as the 3rd century, B.C.,
during the reign of the first Chinese Emperor Ch'in Shih Huang-ti,
the use of *Prana* was part of the secret way to enjoying better
health and better life.

When Buddhism spread throughout China, during the 1st
century A.D., the benefits of "youth breath" were adopted
by many Orientalists. *Prana* was said to be healthful, rejuvenating and the secret of "immortality," to "make the body light"
and also "purify the heart and calm the spirit, so that each
individual may be like Buddha."

When the Hindus used *Prana* and found that they experienced
a feeling of rejuvenation of body and mind, it led the Chinese
to delve into the mysteries of this secret of better health. Chang
Chung-ching, during the Han period, and Hua T'o, who was
said to have discovered anesthesia, wrote extensively about
the healing virtues of "youth breath." The alchemist-physician-
magician, Ko Hung, in the 4th century A.D., prepared a secret
document entitled *Pao P'u-tzu*, in which he offered Taoist
superstition along with sound medical advice on how to use
Prana to cast out demons (infections) and restore good spirits
(youthful health). Other physicians used *Prana* to heal their
patients and reported remarkable benefits. When the Hindu
peoples spread the knowledge of yoga as the secret of eternal
youth and health, *Prana* became a recognized all-natural way
to internal purification of body and mind.

The Hindu Secret of Prana

The Hindus taught a chosen few that *Pranayama* holds the
secret of perpetual youth. *Prana* means "breath," but it includes the youth principles at all levels of consciousness: body,
mind and energy. *Yama* means "restraint," so *Pranayama* means
restraint or *control* of breathing to help regenerate and master
the youth-giving forces at all levels.

The Hindu teaches that as we breathe in, we take in the
youth breath of the Universal Spirit. The suggestion here is
that the nervous system is steadied and calmed so that the

youth currents can flow harmoniously throughout the body, bathing it with nourishment and regeneration.

The Hindu further teaches that in "youth breath," the mind is cleared of external disturbances or aging factors; the mind can now become a source for the Cosmic Life, which offers eternal youth. The Hindu secret is that *Prana* enables you to control your thinking principle, control your body, become "one" with the Cosmic Spirit and, thus, use breath to help regenerate and rejuvenate your entire mind and body. This is part of the Hindu religion and, judging from the amazing longevity as well as perpetual virility of so many centuries-old practitioners, we should note that this *Prana* secret may hold one of the keys to eternal youth.

Special Note: The Orientals explain that *Prana* does not consist of just breathing in and breathing out — this is merely an automatic routine to keep one alive. The Orientals say that for *Prana* to exert its youth benefits, the individual must use his entire nervous system and consciousness. In the following *Prana* secret exercises, you are required to utilize your "inner activity" (*Nei-kung*) and "outer strengthening" (*Ch'iang-chuang-kung*). Together, they form the "way to the preservation of perpetual youth" (*Yang-sheng*). Accordingly, the ancient secret of *Ch'i* (breath, air, youthful energy) becomes known. That is, *Ch'i* restores the vital balance between *yin* and *yang*, thereby rejuvenating the inner organs and also creating a harmonizing balance of body and mind. Once the following *Prana* secrets are properly performed, the internal organs "gradually obey the dictates of the will and their functioning can be controlled," say the ancient writings.

Many Taoists, Buddhists and Hindus have reported that *Prana* offers the transcendental (weightlessness) state so invaluable in helping to replenish and rejuvenate the body and mind. Above all, these secret "youth breath" exercises must be performed *without* strain, *without* impatience, *without* forceful effort; to perform them under stress would be to negate their benefits. Instead, the Hindus offer a 3-step "total relaxation" program that is to precede the subsequent 8-step *Prana* way to perpetual youth.

The Three-Step "Total Relaxation" Hindu Secret

1. Relax Yourself *(Sung-ching Wei Chu).* Let your entire body and mind be cleansed of any influences; your spirit should feel at peace. Relax your muscles as a means of helping to relax your mind and spirit. Let yourself be bathed in an aura of total peace.

2. Contemplate Breathing *(I-ch'i Ho-i).* Focus your entire attention upon your breathing; but breathe gently. The Hindus say that the breathing is *not* work; it is not to be forced. It is to be soothing, gentle and as natural as one's own heartbeat.

3. Feed Yourself Youth Breath *(Lien-yang Hsiang-chien).* As you relax your body and mind, "feed" yourself with the pre-scribed breathing exercises. This creates an interaction of breathing and rejuvenation. Do *not* strain yourself. Strive for a *balance.*

Rejuvenation Benefits of the Three-Step Secret

The Hindus maintain that such preparation helps refresh the body and the mind. Modern science recognizes these reported benefits: the internal organs are rejuvenated, the appetite is refreshed, the blood circulation becomes stimulated. In partic-ular, the cerebral cortex portion of the brain is soothed by the diaphragmatic breathing to create an "air wash" of the brain cells. This reportedly helps nourish the brain cells and helps prevent symptoms of senility.

A Hindu Prescription for Proper Sitting

The Hindus offer this "prescription" for proper sitting as you perform the following *Prana* exercises:
Sit on a base that is firm, but comfortable, such as a folded-over flat blanket or a flat seat cushion. Rest the instep of one foot on the opposite thigh. This is the familiar Yoga position of cross-leggedness on a mat or flat cushion, which helps ease tensions from the body. Fold both hands gently on your lap. Now you should begin to feel relaxed as tensions leave the body and mind and you contemplate the *Prana* "youth breaths," which follow.

Hindu Directions on How to Breathe

You need to breathe naturally — without force. Slowly increase the depth until you feel diaphragmatic inhalation. Breathe through your nose. Focus your eyes and thought on your navel. Your sole thoughts should be upon the words "youth breath" and "peace." Send these same thoughts to all of your body parts as you slowly breathe in and out.

Secret Benefit: In the cross-legged pose, with steady breathing and emphasis upon diaphragmatic inhalation, there is a relaxation of the cerebral cortex. This breathing will also help improve the function of the diaphragm, itself, building resistance to colds, respiratory ailments, allergies and related ailments involving the respiratory tract. In particular, the problem of prolapse of the stomach (or a heavy pot belly) may be eased. The abdomen is pressed upwards by a natural rhythmic exercise as the breathing is performed. The Hindus are known for being lean, with youthfully *flat* stomachs. Regular *Prana* practices do much to help them keep fit and youthful.

The Hindu Secret of "Youth Breath" Prana — In Eight Steps

The perpetual youthfulness of the Hindu, and others in the Orient who follow *Prana,* may well be traced to this 8-step secret, which was once utilized only by a chosen few:

Before You Begin: Remember to follow the 3-step "total relaxation" program and then adopt the proper sitting pose. Once you are relaxed, you can benefit from these eight steps to perpetual youth, according to the Hindu secret of *Prana:*

1. Chewing Exercises. As you keep breathing in and out in gentle motions, pretend that you are chewing. Place the palms of both hands over your ears while the fingers are on the back of your neck. Press your right middle finger with your left index finger. You should feel a gentle soothing sensation. Repeat several times.

Hindus teach that this relieves headaches, promotes better hearing and alerts the mind.

2. Face Right and Look Toward the Left. As you keep breathing in and out in gentle motions, move your head and shoulders toward the right — but gently look toward the left. Keep repeating several times.

This contrasting movement helps liberate tight knots in the back of your head. It also promotes better circulation and helps relax the back muscles to ease that tight knot between the shoulder blades.

3. Move Your Tongue and Swallow. Keep breathing in and out in gentle motions. Now, move your tongue all over your mouth, along your gums from top to bottom. Rub your tongue against your palate; then, start swallowing gently. Repeat several times.

This breathing-swallowing exercise is said to help stimulate a flow of digestive juices. This helps promote youthful digestion and aids in assimilation of nutrients.

4. Gentle Back Rub With Your Palms. Keep breathing in and out in gentle motions. Now warm your palms by rubbing them together. Reach behind to massage both sides of your spinal column, in your lower back, behind your abdomen, over your pelvis. Keep massaging. Keep breathing.

This helps relieve problems of backache, restores better flexibility to the pelvic region and stimulates the entire body.

5. Arms-Outward Extension. Keep breathing in and out in gentle motions. Now tighten your fists. Reach your arms out as far as is comfortable, but keeping them even with your sides. Now, pretend you are pulling something toward yourself. Repeat several times.

This is a combination of respiration and physiotherapy that firms up tissues and cells and also helps straighten out the spinal column, giving better posture.

6. Self-Ventilation. Keep breathing in and out in gentle motions. Now make fists with both hands. Put fists on your chest. Rotate your shoulders and arms backwards. Repeat several times.

This performs a rhythm from within that helps improve the function of the entire respiratory organs and internal systems.

This promotes a Hindu-prescribed "self-ventilation" that is a form of aeration required to help cleanse the body of internal pollution.

7. Palms Upward. Keep breathing in and out in gentle motions. Now reach your arms forward but keep your palms upraised. Slowly bend your forearms until your upraised palms are in front of your face. Repeat several times.

These motions reportedly help create a better functioning of the entire digestive-elimination system because of a rhythmic massage of these vital youth-creating organs. They promote better digestion and better elimination.

8. Muscle Relaxant and Joint Flexibility. Keep breathing in and out in gentle motions. Now slowly stretch out your formerly crossed legs. Very slowly, lower your head in a worshipful manner. Stretch out your arms. Touch your toes. Repeat several times.

This rhythmic movement helps to relax the muscles, loosen up tight joints, guard against distress of arthritis or rheumatism and also boost youthful circulation.

Additional Suggestions: The Hindu teaches that these secrets are effective if performed gently, in a quiet environment. There should be no strain, no effort, no compulsion, no force. Keep on breathing as the exercises are performed from numbers 1 through 8. At the end, the Hindu says there should be a general feeling of youthfulness and vitality. Many have found that daily practice of these eight steps helps guard against illness. It is a form of natural medicine, according to ancient and modern practitioners of the secret therapy of *Prana*.

Modern Science Accepts the Hindu Secret of Youth

Modern Oriental scientists accept the Hindu secret of *Prana*, or "youth breath." They point to the Pavlovian theory of the nervous system. (Ivan Pavlov was a Russian Physiologist, who lived from 1849-1936. He helped explain the purposes of the nervous system and reflex reactions.) The modern Oriental scientists explain that combinations of the preceding respiratory-relaxation exercises help by stimulating the cerebral cortex of the brain into a condition of youthful harmony. When the cerebral cortex is thus stimulated, the entire body falls under healthful control. This strengthens the body's resistance to pathogenic agents (causes of illness and aging). The general condition of youthful health is in a state of equilibrium, or *yin-yang* balance.

The breathing exercises of Prana help strengthen the body's defense mechanism against illness and aging. The physical exercises accompanying *Prana* help stimulate the internal organs and promote better function and regeneration.

Researchers of the physiological clinic at the First Medical Academy in Shanghai note that *breathing in* will help stimulate the sympathetic nervous system, and that *breathing out* will help stimulate the parasympathetic nervous system. They suggest that proper Prana exercises should help heal problems of the autonomic nervous system. While routine breathing does sustain life, it is the combination of breathing with the Prana exercises, followed from 1 through 8, which promotes the harmony that creates youthful health.

How Prana Helped Ease Ulcer Distress

In one reported case, a 28 year-old workman, Chu X. Y., was troubled with a diagnosed duodenal ulcer. He had severe abdominal pains and also experienced waves of nausea. He experienced pain in his back, brought up gastric acid and had fits of giddiness, and he reportedly had a low red blood corpuscle count. He was admitted to the Sixth Municipal Hospital in Shanghai for treatment and was placed on the Prana program.

Healing Begins Promptly. On March 23, immediately upon beginning the Prana breathing program, Chu's physical condition improved. His appetite was better and his lumbar pains subsided. Soon, his abdominal pains ended. On April 5, all symptoms of ailment vanished. Chu's complexion was rosy and his weight was healthier. His red corpuscle count also increased, and X-rays showed that his duodenal ulcer was completely healed. Chu's stomach was no longer painful from pressure. *Within two weeks of Prana breathing, Chu was pronounced cured!* Soon, he left the hospital, feeling young and healthy.

Prana Helps Rejuvenate an "Aging" Stomach

In another reported case, 35 year-old Wei X. Y. complained of experiencing sharp stomach pains after meals. He had a long history of irregular digestion for about 18 years, and he had such strong abdominal and intestinal pains that he applied to the Central Hospital in the Huangfu Region of China for treatment.

Medication Increases Discomfort. At the Central Hospital, he was diagnosed as having a duodenal ulcer and prolapse of the abdomen. He was given medication and, although the pains subsided, he had more discomfort. He could hardly eat; he felt ailing and old.

Prana Exercises Restore Youth to His "Aging" Stomach. Wei then went to the Shanghai Sanatorium for Respiratory Therapy, which offered *Prana* as a traditional healing program. Wei entered the hospital on March 27th. After a thorough examination, he was put on a series of Prana exercises, as described above. Almost immediately, the excess gastric acid was reduced. Wei felt relief and freedom from the stomach pains. On April 2nd, he felt much, much better. On April 14th, less than three weeks of Prana treatment, all pains subsided. His stomach felt youthful, his appetite was good, his weight improved and he showed an increase in red blood corpuscle count. He was healed, thanks to Prana, and all this within three weeks of the "youth-breath" treatment.

According to Liu Kui-chen, M.D., in his *Practice of Respiratory Therapy (Ch'i-kung Liao-fa Shih-chien)*, some 500 patients were successfully healed in the past eight years, using the *Prana* "youth breath" method *without* any medication or drugs. Dr. Kui-chen writes that his staff at the Shanghai Sanatorium makes use of the latest scientific equipment in using this respiratory treatment. It is a combination of the past and the present. The goal is to help establish body harmony, or *yin-yang* balance, using either a few or no drugs at all. Since *Prana* has healed so many people throughout so many centuries, it is reasonable to believe that it works today, in many modern hospitals throughout the Orient.

Prana Rejuvenates Reflex Functions

Modern Oriental and Western physicians note that the internal organs respond to reflexes. They agree that breathing can regulate the pulse and blood pressure, and they also feel that Prana can healthfully rejuvenate the functioning and responding of the internal organs, including the digestive system, heart, liver and kidneys. Prana further promotes a smooth musculature of the blood vessels to facilitate a better blood circulation and oxygenation of the body from head to toe. This is the *Prana* secret of perpetual youth: *Give living air to your body and you have hope for better health, better strength and "forever young" vitality.*

SUMMARY:

1. As far back as the 6th century B.C., the secret of *Prana* was known to a select few who used rhythmic breathing to achieve a feeling of health and perpetual youth.
2. Begin Prana by total relaxation in three easy steps, according to the Hindus. Sit comfortably.
3. In just 30 minutes, you can perform the eight secret Prana breathing exercises that reportedly help promote healing and rejuvenation of body and mind.
4. Chu, a 28 year-old workman, was healed of ulcers by following the Prana method of healing. No other medications were used.
5. Wei, a 35 year-old man, was healed of gastric distress and ulcerated stomach and prolapse of the internal organs through supervised *Prana* treatments, used exclusively. In three weeks, his "aging" stomach was healed and rejuvenated.
6. Modern scientists throughout the world recognize the rejuvenating values of this once-secret Hindu method of perpetual youth.

17

Honey:
Health-Giving Secret
from the Orient

Throughout all of the Orient, including the Middle East, honey has been used as a natural healer for hundreds of centuries. In ancient days, many Orientals would offer honey to the gods in the hopes that this sacred food would strengthen the deities who, in turn, would reward the people with equally good health. The sacred rites of the Babylonians, Assyrians, Phoenicians, Hebrews, Chaldeans, Chinese, Japanese and Indians included the use of honey in all their ceremonies. It was part of their sacred training to prepare a vessel of honey for use in Heaven, and in many Oriental nations, a child was given a jar of honey at his birth, to assure him a life of purity and goodness.

Honey is Regarded as a Love Philter

Many Asiatics regarded honey as an aphrodisiac. They felt it possessed a secret or magical substance that influenced the fertility of women and the virility of men. Middle Eastern folks would use honey in wine at wedding celebrations and it was said that they would become so stimulated that an orgy would ensue. Many claimed that honey was a secret love philter that would prompt an ancient satyriaca (an effulgent sexual em-

207

brace, *ad coitum tentaginem irritantia facientia*). Tradition held that an elixir made with honey would promote a sudden glow of vigor and energy that would turn a weak person into a powerful sexual lover.

The Honey Potion That Promised Rejuvenation

In ancient days, among the Orientals, a simple honey potion that came to be called *mead* was said to offer a feeling of rejuvenation.

This simple recipe calls for boiling three parts water to one part honey over a slow fire until one-third has evaporated. Let it cool. Then sip slowly. This Honey Potion is considered an aphrodisiac by the Middle Eastern peoples, who are forbidden alcoholic beverages by their religion. It is said to promote a feeling of rejuvenation and youthful virility.

This same Honey Potion, or *mead*, is mentioned frequently in the Bible and in many sacred books of India. The Persians claimed that they became rejuvenated when they sipped a mixture of boiled milk and honey in the early hours of the morning, and the followers of Islam also considered honey to be a secret nectar of perpetuating youth.

Throughout India, Persia, Arabia, Assyria, China and Japan, honey was used as a natural medicine — and this is based on more than just religious belief or tradition. In modern science, we have discovered the many secret youth-restoration powers of honey.

The Magic Health-Building Powers of Honey

Honey is one of Nature's golden treasures that cannot be man-made, and it is a source of many substances that help build health. Here are a few of the magic health-building powers of honey:

Honey Contains Seven Digestive Aids. The ancient and modern Orientals enjoyed youthful digestion through eating honey. This magic food contains seven valuable enzymes:
   1. *Invertase* (converts sucrose to dextrose and levulose)
   2. *Diastase* (converts starch to maltose)

3. *Catalase* (decomposes hydrogen peroxide)
4. *Inulase* (converts inulin to levulose)
5. *Aromatic bodies* (terpenes, aldehydes, esters)
6. *Higher substances* (mannitol, dulcitol)
7. *Maltose* (rare energerizers, melezitose)

Honey is a Nutritional Powerhouse of Magic Healers. In addition to its digestive enzymes, honey contains many minerals, seven members of the vitamin B-complex group, vitamin C, dextrins, plant pigments, amino acids, traces of protein, esters (forms of enzymes) and aromatic compounds. Honey contains an average of 17% water, 40% levulose (fruit sugar), 34% dextrose (grape sugar), 2% sucrose, 2% dextrins, and goodly amounts of silica, iron, copper, manganese, chlorine, calcium, potassium, phosphorus, sulfur and magnesium.

Honey Produces Youthful Energy. Since 80% of its composition is natural sugar, honey has energy-producing value. Other sugars must be broken down into simpler sugars by digestive enzymes before they can be absorbed into the bloodstream, but honey has pre-digested sugar, requiring very little enzyme action. Honey creates speedy absorption for youthful energy within a short while after consumption.

Honey is Soothing to the Digestive System. The natural sugars in honey are basically dextrose and levulose (simple sugars that are pre-digested). The benefit here is that these two sugars require little enzymatic-digestive action in order to be absorbed. The Orientals recognize this "instant digestion" of honey and use it to soothe their digestive systems.

Honey is Said to be a Pure Healer. Since bacteria, which sometimes cause illnesses, cannot live in honey, it is said to be a safe and pure healer.

How to Store and Use Honey

Honey should be stored in a dry place because it absorbs and retains moisture. Do not refrigerate it; this may hasten granulation. Honey may be used in place of other sweeteners, and it may be used for sweetening in beverages, both hot and cold.

Oriental Secrets of Healing With Honey

The Orientals used honey for internal rejuvenation and also for external healing. Here are some of their secrets as they were found in various scrolls and forgotten writings:

Constipation: Eat several tablespoons of raw honey, every day.

Diarrhea: Eat boiled honey, which is warm and soothing and reportedly helps relax the intestinal regions.

Magic Breakfast: A popular Oriental "magic breakfast" (said to provide immunity against illness and old age) called for eating honey, onions and bread, every morning.

Inflammation: For external inflammations, apply a poultice of honey and then bandage accordingly. For internal inflammations, go on a one or two-day fast during which nothing is taken except cups of boiled water with honey. Sip the boiled water-honey tonic very slowly.

Sores: The Greek physician, Hippocrates, learned from Orientals about the values of honey. Wrote Hippocrates, "Honey causes warmth, cleans sores and ulcers, softens hard ulcers of the lips, heals carbuncles and running sores." For breathing difficulties, he also recommended honey.

Bronchitis: Dissolve honey in a cup of boiled milk. Sip slowly to ease respiratory distress.

Lifetime Immunity: In a reported case, J. J. H. tells of his grandmother who, as a child, was diagnosed as having consumption and given a short time to live. Someone suggested she try the Oriental secret of lifetime immunity — to drink goat's milk with honey every day. It is reported that this grandmother (when she was a child) began drinking this Oriental tonic every single day. The result is that she lived to the age of 88 and enjoyed lifetime immunity from all illnesses.[1]

Freedom from Illness: M.D.A., a beekeeper, told his physician that he had eaten honey for over 30 years. "I can tell

---

[1]Bodog F. Beck, M.D., and Doree Smedley. *Honey and Your Health* (Dodd, Mead and Company, 1966).

about my own experience and give also observations of other people who use honey exclusively for sweetening. I have never known a beekeeper who had any kind of kidney trouble. They all have a clear complexion, good eyesight and no lameness. Among my friends who eat honey and keep bees, there is no paralysis."[2]

Japanese Sleeping Potion: Mix two tablespoons of honey and the juice of half a lemon in a glass of hot water. Stir vigorously. Sip slowly about an hour before retiring. The Japanese traditionally use this all-natural sleeping potion and enjoy healthful-youthful sleep.

Digestive Tonic: For an all-natural digestive aid, Orientals always dip into the honey pot and enjoy freedom from distress.

Secret Benefit: Honey does not ferment in the stomach. It is an inverted sugar and is speedily absorbed, so there is no risk of a bacterial invasion. The honey flavor also promotes a flow of digestive enzymes.

For Natural Regularity: In the Orient, where patent medicine laxatives were unknown, honey was taken for a natural regularity tonic.

Secret Benefit: Honey has a lubricating benefit. Its natural fatty acid content stimulates peristalsis and helps establish regularity. It also soothes problems of gastric catarrh, hyperacidity, gastric distress and gall bladder unrest. These ailments were totally unknown in the Orient where honey was their natural food and natural medicine.

Hindu Secret of Long Life: The Hindus of India look upon honey as a food and medicine and also a secret of long life. The Hindus drink *madhuparka* (a mixture of honey and curds, or the lumpy portion of cottage cheese) during special ceremonies with the toast, "I drink thee for long life, everlasting health and enjoyment of my years."

Sore Throat: Mix honey, lemon juice and egg white and sip with a spoon. This is said to ease coughing spasms and promote soothing of sore throat distress.

---

[2] Ibid

Skin Rejuvenation: In ancient and modern Persia (now Iran), women have long used a special Persian skin rejuvenator. Combine 1/2 cup barley, one tablespoon of honey and enough egg white to make a thick paste. Apply to the face and let remain up to an hour. Then rinse off with contrasting warm and cold water, finishing with cold water to tighten the pores. This is said to help smooth the skin, soften and erase wrinkles, and bring a colorful glow of youth to the face.

Cleopatra's Beauty Secret: The Mediterranean beauty, Cleopatra, is said to have acquired this secret from caravaners from the Middle East. Mix equal amounts of oatmeal and honey until they become smooth and thick. Apply this to the face as a mask and let it remain up to 15 minutes; then wash off with contrasting warm and cold water; finish with cold water to tighten the pores. It is said that many Oriental women who prize youthful skin use Cleopatra's beauty secret once a day, and their enviably pink youth is proof of the healing benefits of honey.

Oriental Wrinkle-Erase Secret: The equisite, China-doll, pristine purity of the Oriental female's skin is often envied by non-Asiatics. The Oriental female must submit to harsh Asiatic climates and expose herself to strong sun and corrosive winds, but she has been taught to protect herself against the formation of wrinkles by using a traditional beauty secret. It is known as the Oriental wrinkle-erase secret.

Mix the beaten white of one egg with one tablespoon of honey. Spread this over the face and let it remain up to 30 minutes. Wash off with warm water and finish with cold water. The benefit here is that nutrients in the honey are propelled by nutrients in the egg white within the outer layer of the skin. These nutrients burrow beneath the skin surface to promote "plumping up" of the "reservoirs" and thus help maintain firmness, suppleness and youthfulness. This is a traditional Oriental secret used by many lovely Asiatic women, who may look as young as 15, yet be as old as 80, or more!

Rough Red Hands: The lovely hands and the graceful fingers of the Orientals may well be a result of this centuries-old secret remedy: massage rough red hands with a mixture of honey and orange juice. Massage well into the skin and let it remain up to 30 minutes; then rinse off with hot followed by cold water. It is said that nutrients in the honey and the orange juice help replenish the broken cells of the skin and rebuild tissues to overcome the rough redness of chapping.

Hair Growing Secret: The enviable hair of Japanese geisha girls may be traced to a centuries-old secret. It is said that Japanese girls mix several tablespoons of honey with alcohol (about 80 proof, available at most pharmacies), stirring them together. They then massage this remedy into the scalp, let it remain for two hours, then shampoo out thoroughly. It is said that regular use of this honey-alcohol mixture stimulates the hair follicles to grow into luxuriant tresses.

Energy Tonic: Workmen in the Orient are always in need of energy and strength. They often rely upon this simple energy tonic: honey diluted in boiled water, then sipped as the beverage becomes comfortably tepid. Today, many modern Orientals will carry a thermos of this energy tonic, to be sipped as an all-natural pep tonic.

Secret Benefit: Honey is a concentrated and predigested food that is instantly absorbed to produce natural energy. Because of its demulcent effect, rapid assimilation and ability to boost energy without fermentation, this energy tonic is a powerhouse of vitality.

How Honey Helps Heal Arthritis

In a reported situation, J. L. was diagnosed as having problems of arthritis. His doctor put him on an Oriental program — a fruit fast. J. L. was told to eat fresh fruit and honey every day, and nothing else, for about three days. He followed this Oriental program, which was said to promote youthfulness of the limbs and restore flexibility. Within a week, J. L. felt better, his arms and legs became youthful, and the pains in his knees were gone. Now he felt healthfully young, thanks to this simple fruit-honey fast program. He returned to his regular eating program, but occasionally went back on this fruit-honey fasting program for three days a month. His symptoms of arthritis never returned.

Honey Hastens Healing

The Hindus and Chinese will cover scratches, wounds and open sores with thick blobs of honey and let the application remain for several hours. Also, Orientals will use honey in ointments, plasters or concoctions for boils, burns and wounds. It is said that honey is gentle and soothing and helps to ease inflammation, resist putrefaction and promote better healing. It is the Oriental's all-natural first-aid medicine.

Honey — Oriental Medicine From the Bee Hive

To the Oriental, honey is more than a natural sweetner — it is Nature's medicine from the bee hive. Modern science knows that honey has speedily digested natural sugars, and that these sugars are in a pre-digested form, having reached that state through the enzymatic action of the bee's glands.

Natural Alkalizer. If you are troubled with acid indigestion, use honey as a natural alkalizer. It is an alkaline food, containing ingredients similar to those found in fruits, which become alkaline in the system.

Helps Maintain Body Youthfulness. Honey also improves the retention of calcium, which is needed for building the strong nerves and strong bones common to Orientals. Honey boosts the hemoglobin count and uses its good iron and copper supplies to help heal problems of anemia. It helps soothe the kidneys and liver, helps protect against illnesses of the respiratory and digestive tracts, boosts the health of the heart and promotes a balm of relaxation and soothing contentment.

Honey is also the Oriental's best bacteria-destroying natural medicine. When troubled with almost any infection, whether internal or external, the Oriental uses honey. It has helped his ancestors for thousands of years, and it helps him, today. It can help you, too!

HIGHLIGHTS:

1. Honey was used as a youth-health food for thousands of years throughout the Orient. It was said to be a powerful aphrodisiac or love philtre. The Honey Potion, *mead*, easily made in your own kitchen in a few moments, has been used as a "love potion" by many Middle Easterners of the past and the present.
2. Honey contains seven digestive aids, a treasure of magic healing nutrients and energy-producing ingredients, plus instant digestive abilities.
3. Oriental secrets are filled with healing remedies using honey either alone or with other commonly purchased items. These same secret remedies can be used in our modern times.
4. Honey is the Oriental medicine from the bee hive, reportedly promoting a natural alkalizer benefit and helping to maintain body youthfulness from the inside to the outside. Honey *is* youthful health!

18

The Oriental Secrets for Staying Youthfully Slim — Without Dieting

The youthfully slim Orientals know how to remain lean and healthy on nourishing food programs without the need for drastic diets or reducing drugs. A fat Oriental is a rarity, even in our modern times, when so many calorie-rich Western foods have become known in Asiatic countries. The Orientals know that if they follow simple secrets from the past and present, they will be able to enjoy appetite satisfaction and digestive comfort, and still remain youthfully slim.

Oriental women are known for having a curvaceous figures even at advanced ages. If they do gain weight, they know a few secrets on how to control the appetite and gently lose the excess fat. Most important, the Orientals have secrets for reducing that firm up the skin texture and keep it looking smooth and youthful. This is in contrast to many Americans, who lose weight only to discover that they now have flabby, wrinkled folds of flesh covering their skeletal structure. The Orientals know that the body must be nourished while pounds are melting so that the structures *beneath* the skin surface remain firm and smooth. This leads to weight loss *and* youthful skin.

The Little-Known Japanese
"Quick-Slim" Program in Nine Steps

A Japanese physician has prepared a "quick-slim" program, which helps melt pounds in a short time, provided that nine steps are followed faithfully. He has successfully melted pounds from many hundreds of overweight folks from all parts of the world who come to him for his secrets of a "quick-slim" physique, based upon a modern practical application of centuries of secrets from the Orient.

Shichiro Goto, M.D., Professor at Kyushu University in Japan, offers this nine-step program to his overweight patients with the suggestion that they follow it faithfully. No drugs, no exercises, no starvation, no complications — just the faithful serenity of the Oriental temperament and the honest desire to lose weight and benefit with a healthfully slim body with firm, youthful skin texture. Here is Dr. Shichiro Goto's little-known but highly effective Oriental "quick-slim" program in just nine steps:[1]

Step #1. Follow a regular daily schedule to occupy your mind. Avoid mental or physical overwork since this may lead to compulsive eating and a runaway appetite.

Step #2. Give up smoking cigarettes and drinking alcohol.

Step #3. Avoid excessive temperature extremes since this may interfere with body metabolism and lead to the accumulation of fatty deposits in the body. Avoid working in direct, hot sunlight as much as possible, since this may lead to aging of the skin and wrinkled furrows after weight is lost. Heat also takes out valuable moisture from beneath the skin surface, which leads to drying and wrinkling as weight is lost.

Step #4. Your living and working areas should be well-ventilated; your clothes and your bedclothes, too, should be comfortably cool. This helps regulate a soothing body temperature, which favors gentle metabolism and gentle loss of weight.

---

[1]Shichiro Goto, M.D. *A Way to Health and Longevity* (Kyushu University, Japan).

Step #5. Take comfortably cool baths. If possible, give yourself a rubdown with a *cold wet towel* every morning. This helps stimulate sluggish cells beneath the skin and facilitates better metabolism. It also promotes a form of exercise that helps "plump-up" the skin to create firmness.

Step #6. Eat two meals a day, preferably breakfast and then a main meal in the late afternoon. Your foods should be rich in green-leafy vegetables. Eat fresh fish as often as possible. Dr. Goto tells his patients that if they eat sufficient amounts of fish, they should be able to give up eggs and milk, which he feels are fattening. If meat is eaten, Dr. Goto suggests *small* quantities. He advises his patients to *avoid any animal fat in any form!*

Special Secret: Dr. Goto says that if larger amounts of fat-containing meats are eaten, then large supplies of green leafy vegetables should be eaten at the same time. The minerals from the vegetables help neutralize the acidity of the meats and help create an enzymatic digestive action that helps burn up calorie-causing fats.

Step #7. Drink freshly poured water on an empty stomach, particularly upon arising. This helps flush out accumulated wastes and is said to promote better internal balance.

Step #8. With large amounts of vegetables, you should be able to have regular bowel movements. If there is distress, increase your intake of tough, raw, fibrous vegetables. Chew all foods thoroughly before you swallow.

Step #9. Vitamin K, taken as a supplement (with your doctor's approval) is most helpful in maintaining body health while losing weight. This vitamin is found in tomatoes, green-leafy vegetables, kale and whole-grain cereals, as well as natural alfalfa.

According to Dr. Goto, this nine-step "quick-slim" program has helped many overweights melt off unsightly pounds without the need for medication or special appliances. It is simple, but it is healthfully effective for the grateful "forever-slim" folks who tried his program and now enjoy a youthfully slim figure.

The Vitamin That Helps Keep You
Slim and Perpetually Young

A Japanese scientist, M. Kondo, at the University of Tohoku, participated in the creation of the Mishi Health Program, a little-known yet highly effective food plan that helps keep its followers looking and feeling youthfully slim. It is based upon the proper use of a newly discovered nutrient, Vitamin K.

The Slim-Youth Power of Seaweed

Vitamin K is highly concentrated in seaweeds as well as many vegetables. Dr. Kondo found that folks who ate copiously of fresh seaweed (a staple food in the Orient), enjoyed better health, more youthful figures, prolonged endurance and vitality at very advanced ages.

The Japanese are first among all other Oriental nations in harvesting the sea for sea vegetables and sea greens such as seaweed. They eat these as part of their daily and enjoy the benefits of slim youth and vigor.

Magic Reducing Power of Vitamin K.

Oriental researchers have sought to   penetrate the secret "magic reducing power" of Vitamin K, the prime nutrient in seaweed. Modern researchers have reported that Vitamin K regulates the functions of the adrenal glands and also the reticulo-endothelial systems. This offers a natural hormonal-metabolic *balance,* which is able to promote better assimilation of foods. This is also believed to provide a "burning" of fat, which results in the slimming process that gives the Oriental his enviable slim figure. *Vitamin K in seaweed may well be Nature's all-natural reducing food!* Ancient Orientals knew that it worked and modern Oriental scientists know the reasons why it helps keep the body youthfully slim. Thus, it is part of the Oriental way of keeping slim and healthy at the same time.

Seaweed Promotes Magic Rejuvenation

In a reported case, Alan F., age 40, was troubled with overweight. Alan also had seriously high blood pressure and nearly white hair. He had tried one diet after another with little success. Then, he reportedly adjusted his eating habits based upon Dr. Shichiro Goto's nine-step "quick-slim" program — but with *one* decisive improvement. Alan F. started eating raw seaweeds.

Results? Alan slimmed down. He reportedly gained youthfully firm skin and the look and feel of a teen-ager. His white hair darkened and his natural color returned. He thanks the "magic" ingredients in seaweed for helping him to lose weight, enjoy normal blood pressure and also provide him with the restoration of his natural hair color. Now, he reportedly looks much younger than his 40 years.

How to Use Seaweed

Most health stores sell raw seaweed. Use it as a vegetable; add it to your raw vegetable salads. Crush the leaves and sprinkle over raw vegetables as a Vitamin K dressing. Mix seaweed with soy cheese, add to a bowl of natural brown rice and enjoy a healthy meal that is brimming with Vitamin K — the Oriental secret of perpetual slimness and youthful vitality.

The Simple Hawaiian "Slim Bath" That "Melts Fat" From the Body

Joan K. looked much older than her 50 years because of the rolls of fat that accumulated around her throat, on her arms and around her waist, giving her a "spare tire" that she said she could spare very easily but could not get rid of. She had tried many reducing programs, but while some did help her lose weight, the pounds inevitably came back again. Joan K. thought a vacation in Hawaii could take her mind off food.

At a special health spa, she put herself in the hands of traditional Oriental healers. She was put on a low-fat, low-sugar program and given a special "slim bath," which worked miracles. It was this Hawaiian "slim bath" that helped melt fat from her body. Joan K. thought she could actually see the fat being "dissolved" from her throat, middle and thighs. Most important was that she was slim and firm *beneath the skin,* without any hanging folds of flesh, which are often the consequence of reducing. Here is the secret Hawaiian "slim bath" that helped dissolve fat while Joan K. soaked in a tub:

Secret Hawaiian "Slim Bath": In a comfortably warm bath, add handfuls of raw seaweed. Let the seaweed soak in the water. The secret here is that when seaweed is combined with hot water, it has a natural "fat-melting" action on the body. When Joan K. immersed herself into the tub, the seaweed nutrients combined with the hot water, then worked to absorb many excess fluids and fat substances right through the pores of her body. The seaweed bath made her perspire more than just plain hot water, but the difference here is that the electrolyte magnetic action of the seaweed substances "sucked out" fatty accumulations from her body and helped her slim down. In ordinary steam baths, water is drained out, but will return when the person drinks a few glasses of liquids. Seaweed, however, drains out more than water: it drains out toxic wastes and accumulated fat cells. This helps provide a natural slimming down.

This is a secret Hawaiian "slim bath" that you can perform right in your own home. Just obtain seaweed from any health store or herbal pharmacy and let it soak in a tub of hot water. When the water is comfortably warm, immerse yourself and relax in it up to an hour. You might follow Joan K.'s program of one bath a day, every evening. It helped her slim down within eight days. Now, she is youthfully slim and looks much, much younger than her 50 years. She feels much, much younger, too — thanks to the secret Hawaiian "slim bath."

Control Your Appetite With Seaweed

If you are enslaved by a runaway appetite, here's how to control it: *Eat seaweed daily.* The benefit here is that the rich iodine content of seaweed is nourishing for your thyroid gland. Once your thyroid gland gets the iodine from seaweed, it is able to boost a sluggish metabolism (often the cause of overweight), and thus help food get burned up before it can be turned into fat.

The thyroid gland is often the key to successful weight control, and Orientals eat seaweed regularly to keep the thyroid alert and active. Many Europeans and Americans are now using this "secret" of a natural appetite-taming food — seaweed. When the urge to overeat strikes, eat some seaweed! That's what Orientals suggest in our modern times.

How Orientals Enjoy a Sweet Food
That Helps Keep Them Slim

Throughout the Eurasian nations of Iran, Iraq, Syria, Libya and Egypt, it is traditional to eat a natural sweet food — *honey* for more than just health. It has been found to be an effective way to satisfy the appetite and the sweet tooth and also to help keep one looking and feeling youthfully slim. *The ancient Orientals often suggested the eating of honey by itself, not mixed with other foods, as a means of controlling the appetite and helping to melt obesity.*

How Honey Helps Keep You Slim

Even though honey is a concentrated sweet with calories, it can keep you slim, as modern doctors observe. Here's the secret of the slimming power of honey:

Fats and sugars are carbon-containing and energy-providing foods, which metabolize when in contact with oxygen to create vitality. Sugars that contain *more* carbon substances will produce quicker energy. Fats that contain *less* carbon substances and oxygen than sugars are metabolized slower because their benefit is to provide *reserve* energy.

Fats require more oxygen to "set them afire," and their energy is not meant for instant use; but if there is insufficient sugar to keep the fires burning, the system must then use its reserve fat. Therefore, when sugars from honey are taken into the system they cause a speedy combustion. The fats will burn with the help of the oxygen produced by their "flames." In cases of obesity, this helps fat to become burned, or used up through the rapidity of honey-sugar metabolism.

For Orientals who are overweight due to excesses of rich foods, the use of honey is a way to control the appetite, promote internal combustion and thereby facilitate weight loss. Honey can, therefore, be considered the Oriental all-natural appetite-control food!

How To Use Herbs To Wash Out
Excess Weight-Causing Body Water

The use of herbs for healing had been recorded many centuries ago through the use of tablets, scrolls, barks, papyrus and other writing materials. In particular, Orientals have used herbs to act as diuretics, that is, to help eliminate water from the system and thereby help reduce weight. It is known that water-logged tissues may often cause overweight; so Orientals have traditionally used *natural diuretics in the form of herbs.*

Natural Diuretic Herbs

Among the favored herbs used in past and present Oriental cultures are these:

Garlic. Chew a garlic clove; garlic oil is also effective. This helps improve the functions of the kidneys and stimulate water passage. It also helps increase a natural perspiration and self-cleansing through the skin pores.

Black Currant. Steep the leaves in boiling water for one hour; strain out the liquid and sweeten with honey; then sip as a natural diuretic. This helps stimulate profuse perspiration flow.

Boneset. Steep one ounce of this powdered herb in a pint of boiling water and sip as a cup of tea, flavored with honey. This herb helps produce perspiration, promotes removal of wastes from the body and induces natural kidney activation to help cast-off accumulated liquids.

Borage. Steep one ounce of borage leaves in a pint of boiling water and season with honey. Sip slowly. This is said to act as a natural diuretic upon the kidneys.

Couchgrass. Pour a pint of boiling water over one ounce of this powdered herb; then let steep. Sweeten it with honey and sip throughout the day. This offers healthful activation of a sluggish bladder and kidneys, thereby promoting an increase in perspiration and elimination of wastes.

Jewel Weed. Mix one ounce of powdered jewel weed in a pint of boiling water and let it steep; then sweeten with honey. This is said to have a mild purgative effect upon the kidneys, thereby promoting a healthful flow of urine and perspiration.

Where to Buy Herbs: Ask at your local health food store. Most pharmacies carry a wide supply of such herbs.

Seven Oriental Secrets of Eating To Help Remain Slim and Trim

Many modern Orientals manage to maintain a trim figure because they know how to eat. They do not "diet," but they often follow seven Oriental secrets of eating that help them look and feel youthfully slim. Here are these seven secrets, which you can follow right in your own home or when eating out:

1. Chew Slowly. Enjoy every mouthful of food with culinary pleasure. The Oriental is wise; he knows that the longer he chews, the less he will eat. This is the natural way to control overeating.

2. Enjoy Your Food. As you eat, think about your food and eat with great pleasure. Every bite should be filled with the enjoyable anticipation of delicious taste. This helps satisfy your emotions and also helps to prevent overeating.

3. See Your Food. Much appetite control is possible when you look at what you are eating. Satisfy your "eye appetite"; look at your food as you eat it.

4. Taste Your Food. Let the food roll around in your mouth — savor it — enjoy it. The Oriental concentrates on tasting every bit of his food. He satisfies his taste buds with modest portions of food and helps keep himself slim.

5. Food is Nourishment. The Oriental eats nourishing food. If a food has no nutritional value, avoid it. Give up empty, useless, calorie-building foods. All foods should offer you good, tasteful nutrition.

6. Eat in Leisure. You will satisfy your emotional need for food if you eat in leisure. Do not gulp food down for this can leave an emotional gap that spurs the urge for more food.

7. Eat Only When Necessary. The Oriental, traditionally speaking, eats only when he is hungry! He does not eat when he is nervous, bored or tense. If you find yourself psychologically frustrated, don't rush to the refrigerator; find another outlet for your emotions. Food is for necessary nourishment and not for easing of emotional frustration.

The Oriental has a wise saying. "Chew twice as long — get twice the pleasure — eat half the quantity."

As living proof, we see the svelte and curvaceous physiques of Orientals of the past and present. Practical eating customs, wholesome foods and traditional folk remedies all help keep the Oriental looking and feeling youthfully slim.

IN REVIEW:

1. To help yourself become naturally slim, try the little-known but highly effective Japanese "quick-slim" program — nine easy steps to weight control. It is completely natural: no drugs, no exercises, no special foods.
2. A Japanese scientist has discovered that a vitamin found in readily available foods can help keep you slim and perpetually young.
3. Alan F. loses excess weight, controls blood pressure and has reported restoration of hair color through the eating of a "magic" ingredient found in seaweed.
4. Joan K. slims down in a simple Hawaiian "slim bath" that melts fat from the body. It's all natural and it can be done right in your own home.
5. Honey is the Oriental secret of sweetening your way to weight loss.
6. Orientals use natural herbs as diuretics to help wash out waterlogged and weight-building excess tissues.
7. To eat your way to a slim-trim shape, follow the seven secret steps used by many modern and perpetually young Orientals. Enjoy eating while you lose weight.

19

Ancient Herb Secrets
from the Orient for Modern Living

In a tradition dating back some 5000 years, the Orientals have made use of herbs and grasses for healing. Oriental cultures put their trust in Nature and learned that medicinal herbs could provide magical remedies for almost all ailments. The Emperor Shen Nung studied and used such medicinal herbs, and he prepared a compendium of such herbal secrets in his *Pen-ts'ao,* imparting his knowledge only to a privileged few. This collection was said to contain thousands of different herbal medicaments for almost every known ailment of the body and the mind.

In the *Book of Songs* (Shih Ching), another Oriental sage listed even more medicinal herbs and secrets of healing through the use of Nature's grasses. These secrets were accumulated through personal experience, and many promised a "herb of perpetual life" or a "golden pill of youth." Although such secrets may be more mythical than factual, there is some credibility to be found in the promise of perpetual life and youth.

The ancient Orientals wrote with a philosophical-poetical style, and when the healer promised youthful and eternal life, he undoubtedly meant that there were medicinal herbs that could cure illnesses and promote a feeling of health and vigor. This meant that medicinal herbs could give one a life that was free from age-causing illnesses. Noting that many Orientals have lived beyond the century mark, with freedom from diseases, we can recognize the youth-building properties of Oriental herbs.

226

Oriental physicians gathered many secrets from Nature's medicines and would prescribe them to royal or affluent members of society. Pien Ch'ueh, a respected herbal healer, wrote many texts on the secrets of medicinal herbs. Chang Chung-ching, in the 2nd and 3rd, centuries A.D., also told of herbal medicaments that would ease fever, act as a sedative, tone the body or act as a diuretic. A successor, Ko Hung, an alchemist physician in the 4th century A.D., was said to have cured illnesses in many people with the use of medicinal herbs, and the Taoist physician in the 4th century A.D., was said to have cured illnesses in many people with the use of medicinal herbs, and the Taoist physician T'ao Hung-ching, in the 5th and 6th centuries A.D. compiled even more herbal medicaments. This knowledge was gathered by successors in the 7th Century A.D., who prepared the masterful *Pharmacopoeia of Shen-nung,* listing some 844 herbal healers.

Sun Szumiao, a brilliant Taoist doctor who practiced at the start of the Tang Dynasty (618-907 A.D.), was revered as the "King of Medicaments," or *Yao-wang,* because he exerted magic healing with all-natural herbs. His classic work, *A Thousand Ducat Prescriptions* (Ch'ien Ching Fang) is a treasure of herbal healers using grasses as well as foods for healing. He prescribed the use of soy beans *(Wu-tou, Ta-tou)* for building strength and health.

As printing methods became more sophistocated, more works were listed. The brilliant *Li Shih-chen,* who practiced towards the end of the 16th century, listed nearly 2,000 herbal medicines in his *Pharmacopoeia* (Pen-ts'ao Kang-mu). Dr. Li Shih-chen is credited with having compiled thousands of years, worth of health secrets in one volume, which is still being used as a source of perpetual youth through natural herbs and medicaments.

The Oriental's Faith in Nature

The Oriental cultures were the first to take such full advantage of herbal medicines. The people put their faith in Nature and, because medicine (involving drugs or surgery) was used solely by the very wealthy who could afford it, the poorer folks were left to the use of natural and often free medicinal herbs. The Orientals also had a rich flora available, and they took a very early interest in botany. If plants were unavailable, they would import them. (The export-import trade of plants has been carried on for thousands of years throughout the Orient.) This indicates their faith in using natural remedies — right up to the present time.

Herbs Needed Special Harvest Time

The Oriental knowledge of herbal medicine was thousands of years ahead of its time. The true Oriental physician demanded that herbs be harvested at a special time. In particular, herbs harvested by the full moon were said to be the most potent.

Secret Benefit: Certain plants do retain their active healing ingredients for as long as the dew remains moist on their leaves. This dew moisture is found in many herbs that are picked by nightfall. If the plant is allowed to remain in the early sunlight, the dew can become dried-up and the potency can be severly diminished. This is a secret that has modern scientific validity.

How Orientals Use Herbs For Healing

Traditionally, an ailing Oriental would describe his illness to a herbal physician, who would provide him with a herbal remedy. The *secret* of the Oriental physician was in knowing the *form* of the herb to be used for the specific ailment. Here is a chart that had been a secret discovery by the ancient Oriental herbal alchemists:

Liquid Herb Potion — To cleanse the intestines, to stimulate a sluggish blood circulation and to help create a beneficial *yin-yang* balance.

Herbal Pills — To relieve congestion, to remove a cold feeling from the body, to help improve the respiratory system.

Herbal Powders — To ease digestive distress and to help heal problems of constipation or diarrhea.

Warm Herbal Potions — For winter distress such as colds, influenza, bronchial disorders, coughs, sneezes and sniffles.

Cold Herbal Potions — For summertime distress such as heat stroke, heat exhaustion or any affliction involving body heat or body overheating.

When to Take Herbs

Oriental physicians also had these secrets:

1. For chest ailments or for healing any body portion above the chest, take prescribed herbal medicines *after* meals.

2. For digestive ailments or for healing any body portion below the chest, take prescribed herbal medicines early in the morning and on an empty stomach.

3. For relief of illness in either the arms or legs, take prescribed herbal medicines early in the morning and on an empty stomach.

4. For relief of ailments of the bones or joints, take prescribed herbal medicines in the evening, *after* meals.

Quick, Effective Healing Secret. For an illness that has been long in duration, Oriental physicians suggested the use of *liquid* herbal medicaments. For an illness that has come on suddenly, they suggested the use of *powdered* herbal medicaments.

How to Prepare Herbs

For cutting herbs, use wooden tools; do not use metals. For cooking, use earthenware or glass containers, do not use metal utensils. *Suggestion:* Obtain herbs from a health store or herbal pharmacy and ask that they be prepared using the previously described methods. If herbs are ground in mortars, these, too, should be made of wood or glass.

Secrets of the Effective Use of Herbs

Herbs are most potent when the plants are fresh; storage will deplete potency. All parts of the plant are useful; this includes the blossoms, leaves, seeds, roots and fruits. To prepare, you may dry, brown, roast, soak or boil. Again, ask a reliable herbal pharmacist to prepare fresh herbal medicines for your individual use.

Oriental Herbs That You Can Use in Modern Times

Here is a compendium of Oriental medicinal plants. Their English names are given to make it easier for you to obtain them from herbal pharmacies.

Monkshood. This herb soothes problems of fever, colds and coughs and eases bronchial distress. Mix the pulverized root with raw egg white and apply it to the skin surface to help heal swelling, blemishes, "spots" and bruises.

Sweet Flag. Sweet flag helps stabilize the appetite and soothes an inflamed stomach. (Ancient and modern Persians believed that sweet flag acted as an aphrodisiac and intensified sexual vigor).

Cardamom. This plant helps promote energy and soothes conditions of weakness or fever.

Angelica. This herb acts to cleanse the bloodstream of impurities. A poultice made of angelica and applied to hemorrhoids is said to promote healing.

Burdock. Orientals have prescribed this for problems of constipation. External applications are said to heal skin rashes or ulcerous breakouts.

Wormwood. Orientals have used this to help soothe headaches, relax the body and ease symptoms of dizziness.

Tarragon. This aids in the healing of febrile conditions and diarrhea, and also promotes healing of the digestive tract.

Wild Ginger. This helps relieve the symptoms of winter distress, such as nasal congestion and head colds. The root can also be used as a diuretic.

Senna. Senna is an all-natural laxative that helps establish regularity. Orientals have suggested using it in small doses.

Safflower. This helps correct problems of hyperemia or blood congestion; it also helps to relieve intestinal-digestive upset.

Turmeric. This herb helps heal wounds and skin blemishes when applied as a poultice. It also helps correct joint pains and stiffness.

Horsetail. This works as a diaphoretic and also as an expectorant for problems of chronic coughing or bronchial disorders. Horsetail also helps clear up nasal-membrane inflammation, opens up blocked ear channels and eases problems of headaches.

Barrenwort. The Orientals have used this as an aphrodisiac. They felt that it boosted virility, increased fertility, and promoted a youthful feeling of well-being to the entire body and mind.

Fennel. Used to improve and rejuvenate digestion, this plant has also been used to promote a feeling of youthful well-being.

Gentian. Gentian helps strengthen the skeletal system and improve digestion. When externally applied, this herb is said to soothe tired or burning eyes. It has also been used to heal foot disorders.

Licorice. An Oriental, all-natural pain reliever, licorice has been known to help expand the blood vessels, enrich the bloodstream, and relax the digestive system.

Plantain. This herb is said to help rejuvenate the sexual organs, increase sperm production, and bring about increased virility and fertility.
Secret: Plantain contains a mucilage that acts as an emollient to soothe the internal organs. This creates a feeling of youthful contentment, which may rightfully cause increased virility.

Pomegranate. The pomegranate's bark is a prime source of resin, tannin and alkaloids, which have a natural anthelmintic (worm-killing) benefit. The tannin is also said to be soothing for digestive problems. *Tip:* The skin of the tree's root is its most potent medicinal portion.

Buckthorn. An ingredient in buckthorn, known as emodin, is helpful in digestive healing and in toning the entire body.

Figwort. This reportedly helps soothe a sore through and bring down a high fever. It is a natural cough tonic.

Dandelion. This plant helps soothe stomach disorders and eases feverish conditions. It also provides natural detoxification and self-cleansing of the body.

Herbal Healing Secrets From The *PEN-TS'AO KANG-MU*

Here are some herbal healing secrets taken from the brilliant Li Shih-chen in his classic *Pharmacopoeia*. He advised finding

your illness and then using the listed herbs for that particular
ailment — either singly or in combination:

For Heart and Circulation Improvement: asparagus, camphor,
lobelia, mint, figwort.

Natural Diuretics: garlic, shrubby horsetail, spurge, marsh-
mallow, mint, mulberry (leaves and bark of tree), plantain.

Sudorifics (Inducing perspiration): mugwort, shrubby horsetail, dandelion.

Healing Open Sores: aloe, plantain, gardenia.

Natural Cough Remedies: bellflower, angelica, ginseng root.

Styptics: mugwort, peony.

For Muscle Tone: aloe, camphor.

Restoratives: sweet flag, burdock, magnolia, ginseng root,
sesame.

Sedatives: hemp, maidenhair, ginger.

Natural Pain Relievers: aconite, sweet flag, hemp, chrysanth-
emum.

Self-Disinfectants: betel nut, garlic, mugwort.

Antiseptics: garlic, mint.

Anti-Toxics: sesame, birthwort, cherry.

For Healing Digestive Disorders: potatoe, sweet flag, aloe,
angelica, mugwort, camphor, plantain, dandelion.

For Boosting Metabolism: licorice root, asparagus, plantain,
gardenia.

For Soothing Spasms: aconite, hair grass, hemp, angelica,
peony, mint.

To Ease Inflammation: lobelia, figwort, sesame, dandelion.

For Soothing the Nervous System: milkwort, citrus, gardenia.

For Rejuvenating the Endocrine Gland System: milkwort,
citrus, plantain, gardenia, peony.

For Throat Healing: bellflower, edible tulip.

For Kidney Healing: water plantain, mint.

For Relieving Allergies: angelica, mugwort, hemp, mulberry leaves, shrubby horsetail, sesame.

For Preventing Arteriosclerosis: onion, aloe.

To Improve Eyesight: maidenhair tree, ginger.

Ancient Herbs Used in Modern Times

These ancient herbal medicines, prepared by Li Shih-chen, have become part of our modern healing practices. The ancient alchemists' prescriptions have been verified and found to be most effective when prescribed by modern pharmacologists and medicinal and pharmacological journals issued throughout the Orient explain that herbal medicaments are highly effective in our modern world.

Skin Diseases Healed

According to a modern medical journal, 309 patients who suffered from lifelong and almost fatal skin diseases and body sores were cured within nine months. These 309 formerly "hopeless" patients were reportedly cured when Oriental physicians treated them with medicinal herbs. Nothing else had previously worked, but the same medicinal herbs that had been used for thousands of years helped cure these 309 patients and possibly rescue them from early death!

The use of herbs is truly miracle of healing from the past that is effective in modern times.

IN REVIEW:

1. Ancient Orientals promoted healing and youthful rejuvenation through the use of Nature's medicaments and herbs. These formed the basis of modern scientific healing practices.
2. Oriental physicians have suggested how and when to use herbs for effective healing.
3. Oriental herbs are now available for your use.
4. The brilliant Li Shih-chen, in his classic *Pharmacopoeia,* has revealed some of his herbal healing secrets.
5. Some 309 patients who had near-fatal illnesses were cured through herbal treatments in a modern hospital.

20

A Treasury of Oriental Health
Secrets and Folk Medicine

Oriental folk medicine has a long and honorable history, offering some sixty centuries of recorded discoveries. The Orientals have relied upon these health secrets because they have been taught that healing is made possible through the restoration of body harmony, or the yin-yang balance, and that this requires the use of natural healers that are in harmony with the divine Celestial Beings. It has been a tradition of folk medicine to help heal the cause and thereby bring relief of the symptoms.

Many ancient Oriental scholars prepared scrolls, parchments and secret documents offering health secrets and natural folk medicines for a variety of different ailments. These secrets were handed down from one generation to the next and, slowly, some of the secrets were revealed to the general populace, who could then make their own folk medicines using plants, herbs, fruit vegetables, seeds, nuts and other natural foods. More and more methods, formulae and treatments were recorded. Folk medicine eventually spread throughout most of the Orient, the Middle East and the Eurasian countries of the Old World, and although some health secrets depended upon mystical rites and superstitions, *most of the folk physicians were effective healers. They had to be healers in order to survive, for these folk physicians were not rewarded unless they produced positive results.*

234

Out of this necessity was born a treasury of Oriental health secrets and folk medicine. From these long-forgotten and once-secret treasured volumes, we have accumulated some of the most respected all-natural healing methods. These reportedly promoted healing in the past, and they have been effective in modern times, according to recent reports.

Such Oriental health secrets offer a glimpse into the mystical world of ancient medicine. We sincerely hope that these findings can be the start of a journey toward youthful health and natural healing for the reader.

Oriental Heart Tonic

Boil 7 teaspoons of hawthorn berries in a pot of water. Let it steep. Strain (squeeze the berries) and drink this tea as a healthful heart tonic. Some Oriental healers have suggested adding the motherwort herb for more effectiveness. This is said to provide a feeling of comfort to the heart.

For More Youthful Arteries

For problems of hardening of the arteries, folk physicians have suggested the raw juice of a finely grated potato. Sip before breakfast every single morning. For symptoms of arteriosclerosis, it has been suggested that meat eating be given up. Lots of raw fresh vegetables and fruits should be eaten daily. In particular, *fresh cherry juice* can be an important part of the daily diet. The secret benefit here is that cherries are rich in vitamin C and bioflavonoids, which help strengthen the blood vessels and arteries.

For Relief of Arthritis

Daily seaweed baths, using thick clumps of available sea vegetables, reportedly ease arthritic pains. The secret here is that the water should be very warm so that its heat can absorb the elements of the seaweed. The heat can then penetrate into the body to stimulate metabolism, increase the intake of oxygen, cause free-flowing perspiration and enable the surface vessels to dilate. This reportedly helps to regulate the blood pressure.

Epsom Salts Bath: This is a mixture of the old and new in Oriental and Eurasian healing. Let one pound of Epsom salts dissolve in the bath water. Soak yourself in the comfortably warm tub and remain there for up to 20 minutes. Then rinse off in tepid water, towel dry and relax in bed for an hour.

Pine Needle Bath: Place one pound of dried pine needle leaves (also known as Birch leaves) in a cotton bag. Boil the bag in two gallons of water up to 30 minutes. Pour this water, together with the bag, into a hot tub of water. Soak in this tub for at least 30 minutes. Such baths are said to help limber up tight or arthritic-like joints.

Liniment for Aching Limbs

For problems of aching joints or rheumatic distress, Oriental folk physicians have prescribed this homemade liniment. Combine one part lanolin with two parts top-quality olive oil and place in a glass jar. Close tightly. Let this stand for up to 24 hours. There is no need to shake the jar. Now, brush this liniment *lightly* on the aching parts. Cover with gauze and let it remain on the affected region. Daily changes are suggested.

An Ointment to Reduce Swelling

When Orientals were troubled with arthritic-like swelling, the natural folk physician often prepared this ointment: Mix 1 pound of salt with 1/2 pound of dry mustard. Add just enough paraffin to create a heavy cream. Let it remain in a glass jar (covered tightly) overnight, at room temperature. After this, you may use the ointment. Just rub it into the swollen region until it becomes absorbed and let it remain for 24 hours; then wash it off with warm water. Repeat this treatment regularly until the pain and swelling subside.

Self-Rubdown Muscle Relaxant

For tight or twisted muscles, Oriental folk physicians had this secret remedy. Combine equal portions of horseradish juice with pure paraffin. Mix until combined. Now rub and rub and rub onto the aching muscular region. Use gentle but firm finger pressure. This is said to help ease muscular spasms and joint aches. *Tip:* You may bandage the afflicted region with woolen cloths to keep it warm overnight.

Stomach Tonic

Boil one tablespoon of dry cornsilk (available at most herbal pharmacies) in water for 15 minutes. Flavor with honey and drink as a tea. Several cups of this herbal stomach tonic daily are reportedly effective in easing digestive distress.

For Asthma-Allergy Disorders

Oriental physicians ordered their asthmatic patients to give up meat. Starches were also taboo. They were told to eat lots of fresh fruits and raw, fresh vegetables. This reportedly gave them a powerhouse of vitamin C, which rebuilt the respiratory-nasal tracts and helped resist sensitivities to dust. These secret folk remedies were then prescribed to relieve asthma-allergy disorders.

Ginger Tea: Wash, peel and grate ginger. Let it steep in boiled water and add honey for flavoring. Drink several cups throughout the day.

Secret Nasal De-Congestant: Grate 1/2 pound of fresh horseradish and add the juice of two lemons. Keep this thick mass in a glass jar, in a cold place. Take 1/2 teaspoon twice a day — mornings and at noontime. *Do not drink any liquids for one hour before or after taking this Secret Nasal De-Congestant.* This brings on a natural release of accumulations that plague the breathing apparatus of the allergy victim.

Natural Inhaler: Place pine needles and cones in a kettle filled with water. Let it boil. Now cover your head, hold your face over the kettle and breathe in the steam from this herbal infusion. About 30 minutes' treatment is said to help relieve nasal congestion and ease throat constrictions.

To Prevent Skin Blemishes

For problems of acne, boils and scales, Oriental folk healers have suggested applying fresh, finely grated carrots to the wounds. Bandage and change several times daily. This is said to help promote natural healing and also reduce swelling.

Exercise for Relief of Constipation

To promote liberation from intestinal-digestive clogging, many Oriental and Eurasian folk physicians offered this simple but reportedly effective three-step exercise to relieve constipation:

1. While lying in bed, lift your body up and down in a sitting position but *do not use your arms.* Put pressure on your abdomen. Repeat up to 25 times in the morning.

2. Stand firm on the floor. Place hands on your hips. Gently lower yourself into a squatting position. Repeat up to 25 times.

3. Lie down. Massage your stomach with your arm, which should be wrapped in a towel. Massage from your rib cage down to your pelvic bones in all directions. Use very little pressure. Repeat this up to 15 minutes. It is reported that these exercises help loosen intestinal-digestive congestion and promote natural regularity.

Natural Laxatives

Oriental folk physicians have suggested that all-natural laxatives be taken in the morning. Usually, *one* of these secret remedies, taken daily, can promote relief within a few days.

Cabbage Juice: Drink two glasses of freshly prepared cabbage juice every morning *before* breakfast.

Oat Tonic: Boil two tablespoons of oats in a glass of water for 5 minutes; then let it cool. Drink this before breakfast.

Cucumber-Kelp Elixir: Soak fresh cucumbers in kelp or salt water for several hours. Drink the liquid in the morning before breakfast.

Tibetan Tonic: Fill a bottle with fresh vegetable juice. Add one finely cut onion. Let this remain in a warm place overnight; then strain. Use just two teaspoons of this Tibetan tonic in a glass of cold water, twice daily, before meals.

Prune-Lemon Potion: Soak natural, sun-dried prunes overnight in lemon juice, honey and boiled water. Use a glass jar; do not use metal utensils. The next morning, drink one glass per hour, prior to breakfast. Eat the prunes with soured milk or yogurt.

Diabetic Diet

Oriental folk physicians have recognized symptoms of diabetes and reported a simple diet that is said to be healthful and beneficial. It consists of a one week program and calls for the eating of raw vegetables throughout the week. Fat-trimmed meats and fish are allowed and the liberal use of oils is also part of the plan. *Taboo* are chestnuts, cherries, plums, grapes, bread, rice, cereals, peas, raisins, sugar in any form and alcoholic beverages of any sort. *Beverages* should consist of herbal teas, skim milk and buttermilk. Oriental healers have reported examples of healing among their diabetic patients with this one week program. Some patients followed it for a month and were reportedly relieved of the symptoms of diabetes.

To Relieve Diarrhea

Soak dry rye bread in slightly boiled water for 15 minutes: then sip the water slowly. Several such cups, throughout the day, have reportedly eased problems of diarrhea within 24 hours.

To Ease Colitis

Go on a three-day fast during which time meat and eggs are restricted. The diet should consist of milk, whole-grain cereals, softly boiled vegetables and mashed potatoes with butter. Several glasses of carrot juice daily are also recommended by Oriental folk doctors.

Stomach Soothing Elixir: Mix sage and camomile herbs. Use 1 teaspoonful of the herb to a glass of water. Boil for 15 minutes; then strain and season with honey. Sip the liquid slowly. Several cups daily of this stomach soothing elixir are said to calm digestive unrest.

To Alleviate Stomach Gas

Put 1 teaspoonful of anise seeds and 1 teaspoonful of honey in a glass of water. Boil for ten minutes. Cool. Strain. Sip slowly.

Dill Remedy: Boil a teaspoonful of dill seeds in a cup of water for about 15 minutes; then strain. Drink this whenever there is a feeling of gas in the stomach.

To Ease Heartburn

Several cups of goat's milk, taken throughout the day, are said to provide relief of this gastrointestinal disorder. Other Oriental doctor-prescribed remedies call for eating raw, fresh peas. Another highly recommended Oriental remedy for heart-burn is to eat a bowl of whole-wheat buckwheat cereal (sold at most health stores) for breakfast, every morning.

To Improve the Kidneys

Boil one tablespoonful of flaxseeds in a glass of water for 5 minutes. Let it cool; then strain. Add lemon juice (but no honey). Drink a glass of this kidney-rejuvenating tonic every day. Orientals have also recommended these herbs for helping to cleanse, heal and invigorate the kidneys: parsley, dandelion, sweetbrier berries, auricula (primrose) and hemp seeds. Use these singly or in a combination tea.

Liver Cleansing Agent

Even in ancient times, it was recognized that one secret of youthful health was in having a clean liver. Several Oriental doctor-prescribed liver cleansing remedies include:

Beat Juice: Drink one cup of beet juice a day.

Dill Juice: Liquify equal amounts of dill pickles and tomatoes and drink daily.

Berry Tea: Steep the leaves and stems of strawberries in boiled water. Drink several glasses of this berry tea throughout the day.

For Gall Bladder Relief

For problems of the gall bladder, Oriental physicians have prescribed this treatment:

1. Use a laxative to cleanse the bowels.
2. Eliminate all solid foods for one week.
3. Daily, drink at least 5 cups of boiled water (comfortably tepid) to which has been added the juice of one lemon for each cup.
4. Daily, drink raw vegetable juices. Highly recommended are mixtures of carrot, beet and cucumber juices.
5. Remain in bed and rest for as long as possible.
6. Cooperate with your physician.

Oriental folk healers have reported that their patients enjoyed gall bladder relief under this program when followed for just six or seven days.

To Ease Bladder Irritation

Eurasian folk physicians have urged the daily use of any type of oil to ease gall bladder distress.

Nerve Relaxant

A daily rubdown with cool salted water is said to help ease the nervous system. Soaking in a salted tub is also considered an effective, all-natural nerve relaxant. Water should be tepid, at first; then gradually made cooler.

To Shrink Hemorrhoids

All-natural, folk doctor-prescribed suppositories have been made of fresh potatoes and applied to the afflicted region to be retained throughout the day. Another Eurasian suppository is the application of ice. The secret here is to let the ice remain for 30 seconds at first and gradually increase the time up to 90 seconds. One application a day should suffice, and when the hemorrhoids become eased, cold water compresses are suggested until total healing is achieved.

To Reduce High Blood Pressure

Folk doctors have suggested the elimination of fatty meats and starchy foods. The diet should consist of lots of fresh fruits and vegetables, no spices, no salts, no alcohol and no tobacco. Doctors have further prescribed eating garlic daily. Another all-natural "medicine" to bring down high blood pressure is to boil the peelings of potatoes (organic and unsprayed) in a pint of water. Boil for 15 minutes, cool and strain. Two cups daily should suffice.

To Relieve Colds, Sniffles and Coughs

For winter ailments (the winters in regions of the Orient can be most severe), here are some reported natural healers for these cold problems.

1. Press out the juice of grated black horseradish. Mix 1 quart of juice with 1 pound of honey. Take just 2 tablespoonfuls before each meal and before retiring at night. This is said to help heal cold symptoms.

2. Boil 1 pound of bran in 2 quarts of water. Add honey to taste. Drink throughout the day. This is said to ease sore throat.

3. Put several sun-dried figs in a glass of milk. Boil, and let stand for an hour; then warm up again. Drink this while it is comfortably hot. This is said to soothe sniffles and coughs.

4. Combine equal amounts of barley, oats and rye and boil in water or milk. Drink this as a beverage throughout the day. This reportedly helps soothe throat soreness and coughing spasms.

5. For a chest rub, mix 2 parts vegetable oil and 1 part spirits of ammonia (available at herbal pharmacies). Rub into the chest at night for speedy relief.

To Relieve Sciatica

Many Eurasian folk physicians, influenced by the Finnish bath houses, have suggested the application of birch buds and leaves to areas plagued by sciatica. The folk physicians have also suggested soaking comfortably hot bath water to which some eucalyptus essence or oil has been added. They have also recommended massaging with oil regularly.

To Ease Sinusitis

Folk physicians have suggested that sinus sufferers should abstain from all dairy products and take comfortably warm baths daily, breathing in the vapors. A Eurasian prescription calls for the mixing of grated horseradish with lemon juice in a thick sauce. One teaspoonful twice daily (mornings and afternoon) is said to bring relief from nasal congestion. No food or liquid should be taken for one hour before or after this Eurasian home prescription.

For Treatment of Skin Burns

For simple burns, folk physicians have recommended smearing a combination of raw egg yolk and raw egg white over the affected region, followed by the application of alcohol. A healing film forms over the burned region, thus easing the pain and promoting better healing.

Little-Known Secret: If the throat is burned by swallowing a hot beverage, a little-known, secret remedy calls for sipping water to which some egg white has been added. Sip this slowly for relief of a burned throat.

To Treat Sunburn or Windburn

Smear the yolk of one raw egg over the affected area and let it dry. After 30 minutes, wash off with soap and water. This is reportedly effective in easing the burn and restoring softness to the skin.

To Treat Strained or Sore Muscles

Here are two reported folk remedies using compresses.

1. Make a compress of hot fresh milk and apply it to the affected region. Change several times daily.

2. Make a compress of a mixture of grated onion and granulated sugar and apply to the affected region. This is said to be very soothing to pulled tendons or ligaments.

Ear Wash

Hot milk and flaxseed oil (or any available oil) can be soothing as an ear wash, according to Oriental folk doctors.

For Skin Rejuventaion

Apply fresh milk to the skin, rubbing it dry; or, use cold, strong tea (unsweetened) as a rubbing tonic on the skin. Very lovely Oriental ladies have a secret skin rejuvenator — they rub the face with a freshly cut tomato or an overripe yellow cucumber. Do not wash for several hours. When you do wash, use sparkling cold water. This helps rejuvenate the skin, tighten the pores, and give you the look and feel of youth.

Many Orientals have been able to enjoy long, youthful lives because of the wisdom of their folk physicians during some 60 centuries of so-called "unsophisticated" or "unscientific" medical practices. Today, there is a rebirth of interest in folk medicine. Modern medical treatments use such natural methods as hydrotherapy, heliotherapy, exercise, various forms of physiotherapy, massage and plants for healing.

In so doing, we have bridged the gap between East and West: we have drawn from their secrets and they have drawn from ours. It is hoped that, some day, this treasury of knowledge will be able to provide youthful health and happiness for all. Indeed, this was the vow made centuries ago by ancient Oriental physicians.

Index

A

A Thousand Ducat Prescriptions, 58, 186, 227
Abkhasians, forever-young secrets from, 86-92
  history of, 86-87
  longevity as rule, 87
  secrets, all-natural, 87-92
  vitality at advanced age, 87
Absinthe, 183
Acacia, 180
Acupuncture, finger-pressure, 93-103
  (*see also* Shiatsu)
Agar agar as natural laxative, 48, 180
"Aging" stomach, prana and, 205
Alcohol, fruits as help in easing urge for, 151
Algae, 48-49
Alkalizer, natural, honey as, 214
Aloes, 180
American College of Angiology, 171*n*
An-mo, 185-196 (*see also* Reflexology)
Ancient Mysteries, 32
Anemia, help for from apples, 148
Anise, 181
Aphrodisiac, ginseng as, 116
Appetite, control of with seaweed, 221-222
Apple, internal cleansing action of, 61-63
  for "knotted stomach," 62-63
  Persian stomach tonic, 62
Apple as youth fruit of Hawaiians, 147-148
  for anemia, 148
  Polynesian digestive tonic, 147-148
  for stomach upset, 147

Arms, aching, limbering up of with shiatsu, 100-102
Arms, eight steps to "forever-young," 193-195
Arnold, Sir Edwin, 117
Aromatic bitters as ingredient of ginseng, 126
Arteries, healthy, medicine for, 235
Artery-washing, Oriental method of, 168-170
  oils, secret powers of, 169-170
Arthritis, ease of from ocean bathing, 105-107
Arthritis, relief of, 235-236
  help of honey in healing, 213-214
Arthritis stiffness, ocean plants and, 53-54
Asafetida, 181
Asthma-allergy disorders, medicine for, 237
Autolysis of liver, 41-42

B

B-complex vitamins, rice as source of, 72
Backache, shiatsu programs to relieve, 98-100
Balm, 181
Banana as fruit with rejuvenation powers, 145-147
  prescription, secret, 146
Barley brew, digestive healing of, 59-61
  barley bun, 61
Beck, Bodog F., 210*n*
Benefits to Americans of Oriental health secrets, 17-31
Benne, 181

Berries as purification tonic, 66-67
Berry juice fast, 35
Black currant as diuretic herb, 223
Bladder irritation, relief from, 241
Blood pressure, high, reducing, 241
Blood pressure, regulation of by controlled Oriental rice diet, 70-85
(see also Rice diet)
Blood pressure, yoga posture and, 171-172
Blueberries as purification tonic, 66-67
Bodhidharma, 193
Body water, herbs to wash out, 223-224
Boneset as diuretic herb, 223
Book, secret, of plant healers, 56-58
Book of Medicaments of Shen-Nung, 186
Book of the Pulse, 186
Book of Songs, 64, 116, 226
Borage as diuretic herb, 223
Breathing, directions for, 201
"youth breath" prana, eight steps for, 201-203
Bromelain enzyme in pineapple, 149
Brown rice as most perfectly balanced yin-yang food, 29, 70-85
Burdock, 181-182
Burns, relief of, 242

C

Calcium, rice as source of, 72
Carrots for digestive healing, 65-66
Cause of physical disturbance, curing first, 17-18

Cell regeneration through Gotu Kola, 178-180
Chang Chung-ching, 57, 227
Chang-Tu University, 177
Chernych, Dr. S.N., 119
Chewing, careful, essential to yin-yang balance, 23
Chinese Book of Poetry, 47
Chou Inscription on the Technique of Breathing, 197n
Cinnamon, 182
Cleopatra's beauty secret, 110, 212
Clove cocktail, Tibetan, 68-69
Cloves, 182

Cold-water soak for youthful skin, 137
Colds, sniffles and coughs, relief of, 241-242
Colitis, relief of, 239
Common people, good health of, 19
Constipation, relief of, 237-238
Controlled fasting, 85
Cooking rice, Oriental way of, 74-75
Corn remedy, lemon as natural, 64
Couchgrass as diuretic herb, 223
Cucumbers, raw, as liver rejuvenation food, 42
Currant, black, as diuretic herb, 223
Cyclopedia Dictionary of Medical Botany, 119

D

Diabetic diet, 238-239
Diarrhea, medicine to relieve, 239
Digestive aids in honey, 208-209
Digestive healing, use of plants for, 56-69 (see also Plants, use of for digestive healing)
Diuretic herbs, 223-224
Doctors, Oriental, political appointment of, 18-19
Duke University, 73

E

Ear wash, 243
Eating, seven Oriental secrets of, 224-225
Encyclopedia of the Emperor Tai Tsung, 116
Enzymes in ginseng, 126-127
Ergot, 182
Essenes, 33
Eternal youth cult created by Tibetans, 175
Exercises of skin, 135

F

Face-lift, herbal, 134
Family secrets, rise of, 19-20
Fasting, controlled, 85
Fasting programs, ten rice, 75-85
Fasting, Oriental use of, 32-43
herbal tea fast, 39-41

(Fasting, Oriental use of, *cont.*)
  history of, 32-34
  interpretation, modern, 38-39
  liver rejuvenation program, 41-43
    autolysis, 41-42
    benefits of, 42-43
    and cucumbers, raw, 42
    "Mediterranean fast," how to use
      yourself, 35-36
      berry juice fast, 35
      raw vegetable juice fast, 36
    rejuvenation, traditional method of,
      32-34
    reason for, 37
    rules for, 36-37
Finger-pressure acupuncture, 93-103
    (*see also* Shiatsu)
Fish, fresh, 50-51
Fish oils, benefits of, 49-50
  for rejuvenation of heart, 165
  secret power of, 169
Fo-ti-tieng as "elixir of life," 177-178
Folk medicine, treasury of secrets of,
    234-243
  for arteries, more healthful, 235
  arthritis, relief of, 235-236
  for asthma-allergy disorders, 237
  for bladder irritation, 241
  blood pressure, high, reduction of,
    241
  for burns, skin, 242
  for colds, sniffles and coughs, 241-242
  colitis, 239
  constipation, relief of, 237-238
  diabetic diet, 238-239
  for diarrhea, 239
  ear wash, 243
  for gall bladder relief, 240
  heart tonic, 235
  for heartburn, 239-240
  kidneys, improvement of, 240
  laxatives, natural, 238
  liniment for aching limbs, 236
  liver-cleansing agent, 240
  nerve relaxant, 241
  to reduce swelling, ointment, 236
  for sciatica, 242
  self-rubdown muscle relaxant, 236
  for shrinking of hemorrhoids, 241
  for sinusitis, easing of, 242

(Folk medicine, secrets of, *cont.*)
  for skin blemishes, 237
  skin rejuvenation, 243
  for stomach gas, 239
  stomach tonic, 237
  for strained or sore muscles, 243
  for sunburn or windburn, 243
Foods, help of to regulate yin-yang
    balance, 21-25
  secrets, twelve, 21-24
  yang, basic, 24-25
  yin, basic, 24
Foot disorders, use of lemon for, 63-64
"Fountain-of-youth" cocktail, 44-46
"Fruits of passion," juniper berry as,
    182
Fruits, Hawaiian, to rejuvenate digestive
    system, 139-152
  apple, 147-148
    for anemia, 148
    Polynesian digestive tonic, 147-148
    for stomach upset, 147
  banana, 145-147
    prescription, secret, 146
  benefits of, 150-151
  to ease urge for tobacco or alcohol,
    151
  melon, 149-150
  papaya, 140-144
    buying, 144
    health benefits, four, 140-141
    juice for intestinal rejuvenation, 143
    to tenderize meats, 144
    U.S. government praise, 141
    use of by Hawaiians, 141-142
    using, 144
  pineapple, 149

G

Gall bladder relief, 240
Gandhi, Mahatma, 23
Garlic as diuretic herb, 223
General Compendium of Remedies, 58
Ginseng, Korean, as magic herb for
    sexual power, 114-128
  American report, 118
  as aphrodisiac, 116
  case histories, person, 119-120
  harvesting tradition of, 115

(Ginseng, Korean, *cont.*)
  health benefits of, 116-117
  history of, 114-116
  ingredients, secret, 125-126
  of man's shape, 114-115, 117
  meaning of name of, 115
  modern interpretation of, 126-127
  normalization as main benefit, 124
  for perpetual vitality, 124
  references, literary, 116
  rejuvenation, secret formulae for,
      124-125
  Soviet Union acclaim, 118-119
  use, easy ways of, 123
  varieties of, 121-122
  where to buy, 122-123
Ginseng and Other Medicinal Plants,
    120
Goto, Shichiro, 217, 217*n*
Gotu Kola to renew cells and tissues,
    178-180
Gum acacia, 180

H

Haas, M.P., 145*n*
Haas, S.V., 145*n*
Hair, healthy, from ocean bathing, 105
  secrets for, 129-138 (*see also* Skin
      and hair)
Harding, Dr. A.R., 120-121
Harvieu, Father, 94
Hawaiian fruits to rejuvenate digestive
    system, 139-152 (*see also* Fruits,
        Hawaiian)
Hawaiian "slim bath," 220-221
Headaches, relief of through reflex-
    ology, 190-191
"Healing harmony" as basis of Oriental
    healing system, 18
Heart, toning for health and youth,
    164-173
  artery-washing, 168-170
    oils, secret powers of, 169-170
  differences in fats, 167-168
  plant or fish oils, rejuvenation by,
      165
  "right" fats, 167
  "wrong" fats, 167
  yoga breathing exercise, 170-173

(Heart, toning, health and youth, *cont.*)
  and blood pressure, 171-172
  posture, best, 172
  secrets, two, 172-173
Heart tonic, Oriental, 235
Heartburn, relief of, 239-240
Helmut, Wilhelm, 197*n*
Hemorrhoids, shrinking of, 241
Herbal tea fast, 39-41
Herb secrets, ancient, for modern living,
    226-233
  compendium of, 230-231
  faith in nature of Oriental, 227-228
  harvest time for, special, 228
  healing secrets, *Pen-ts'ao kang mu*, 231
  illnesses, list of for herbal treatment,
      232-233
  preparing, 229
  secrets of, effective use of, 229
  for skin diseases, 233
  use of for healing, 228
  when to take, 229
Herbs, Tibetan, healing power of,
    174-184
  acacia, 180
  agar, 180
  aloes, 180
  anise, 181
  asafetida, 181
  balm, 181
  benne, 181
  burdock, 181-182
  cinnamon, 182
  cloves, 182
  cult of eternal youth created, 175
  ergot, 182
  Fo-ti-tieng, 177-178
  Gotu Kola for cell and tissue reju-
      venation, 178-180
  horehound, 182
  hyssop, 182
  juniper berry, 182
  purchasing, 183
  sarsaparilla, 183
  tansy, 183
  wormwood, 183
  writings, early Oriental, 176-177
Herbs as help in healing allergic
    symptoms, 40-41
Hewitt, Edward R., 156, 156*n*

Hippocrates, 210
History of the Late Han Dynasty, 116
Honey, 207-215
    as alkalizer, 214
    for arthritis, 213-214
    healing with, 210-214
    health-building powers of, 208-209
    as love philter, 207-208
    mead, 208
    as medicine from bee-hive, 214
    potion promising rejuvenation, 208
    storing and using, 209
Honey to keep you slim, 222
Honey and Your Health, 210n
Horehound, 182
Hua T'o, 57
Huang-ti nei ching, Emperor, 20
Hyssop, 182

I

Illnesses, list of for herbal treatment,
    232-233
Imperial Encyclopedia, 116
Infection, ginseng helps body resist, 124
International College of Angiology, 171n
Iodine cocktail, 45-46
Iodine replacement as key to easing of
    arthritic pain, 106
Isiduka, Dr. Sagen, 25-26

J

Jesuits of the Scientific Mission, 94
Jewel weed as diuretic herb, 223-224
Juniper berry, 182

K

Kelp as "magic" ingredient of iodine
    cocktail, 45-46
    powder, 47-48
Kempner, Dr. Walter, 73
Kidneys, improvement in, 240
"Knotted stomach," apple as remedy
    for, 62-63
Ko Hung, 186, 198, 227
Kondo, M., 219
Kourennoff, Paul M., 118, 119
Kui-chen, Liu, 205

Kung, Dr. Tsang, 39-40
Kyushu University, 217

L

Laxatives, natural, 238
Lecithin as "magic" ingredient of soy-
    bean, 154-156 (*see also* Soybeans)
Legs, eight-step way to "forever-young,"
    193-195
Lemon, use of for natural rejuvenation,
    132-134
    for foot disorders, 63-64
    for throat disorders, 63
Li Chung Yun, 177
Li Shih-chen, 58, 66, 116, 176, 227
Light of Asia, The, 117
Liniment for aching limbs, 236
Liver-cleansing agent, 240
"Liver rejuvenation" program, 41-43
    autolysis, 41-42
    benefits of, 42-43
    and cucumbers, raw, 42
Longevity as rule with Abkhasians, 87
Love philter, honey as, 207-208
Lubricating effect of honey, 211

M

Macrobiotic diet healing, 25-30
    examples, 28-30
    interpretation, modern scientific,
    26-28
    secrets, seven basic, 26-28
Mead, 208
"Meat without a bone," soybean as, 154
Medicine, all-natural, honey as, 214
"Mediterranean fast," how to use in
    your own home, 35-36
    berry juice fast, 35
    raw vegetable juice fast, 36
    rules for, 36-37
Melon as digestive aid, 149-150
"Melon of health," 140-144 (*see also*
    Papaya as natural fruit medicine)
Metabolic action, freeing of by fasting,
    38-39
Milk, soybean, 161
Minerals, rice as source of, 72
Minkuo University, 177

Mishi Health Program, 219
Motions of reflexology, eight, 187-189
Muscle relaxant, self-rubdown, 236
Muscles, treatment of strained or sore, 243

N

Natural Oriental folk-healers more
    effective than doctors, 18-19
Naturalness of food, importance of, 22
Nature, faith of Orientals in, 227-228
Needham, Joseph, 197n
Nei Ching, 176
Nerve relaxant, 241
Network of Nerves and Vessels, 66
"Newaree," 70-71

O

Oceans, secrets of Oriental vitality
    from, 44-55
  agar agar, 48
  algae, 48-49
  and arthritis stiffness, 53-54
  fish oils, 49-50
    youth oil elixir, 50
  "fountain-of-youth" cocktail, 44-46
  fresh fish, 50-51
  kelp powder, 47-48
  sea plants, 47
  vigor tonic, how to make, 48
  youth-building power of sea foods,
      51-53
    plankton as "complete" food, 52
Ogolevec, C.S., 119
Ohsawa, Dr. George, 26
Oils, secret power of, 169-170
Oils, volatile, as ingredient of ginseng,
    126
Organic foods essential, 22-24
Oriental Health Secrets, 119

P

Penacin as ingredient of ginseng, 126
Pao P'u-tzu, 186, 198
Papaya as natural fruit medicine,
    140-144
  buying, 144

(Papaya as natural fruit medicine, cont.)
  health benefits, four, 140-141
  juice for intestinal rejuvenation, 143
  to tenderize meats, 144
  U.S. government praise, 141
  use of by Hawaiians, 141-142
  using, 144
Pavlov, Ivan, 203
Pearled barley, digestive healing of,
    59-61
Pectin as all-natural medicine, 63
Pen-ts'ao Kang-mu, 58, 116, 176, 226
"Perfect food," reason for consideration
    of soybean as, 156-157
Persian stomach tonic, 62
Pharmacopoeia of Shen Nung, 56-57,
    116, 176, 227
Pien Ch'ueh, 57, 227
Pineapple for youthful digestion, 149
Plankton, consideration of as "complete"
    food, 51-52
Plant oils, secret power of, 169-170
  for rejuvenation of heart, 165
Plants, use of for digestive healing, 56-69
  apple, internal cleansing action of,
      61-63
    Persian stomach tonic, 62
  berries as purification tonic, 66-67
  book, secret, 56-58
  carrots, 65-66
  how they work, 58-61
    barley brew, 59-61
    barley bun, 61
  lemon for throat disorders, 63
    for foot disorders, 63-64
  potato, 64-65
  radishes, 65
  Tibetan clove cocktail, 68-69
Polynesian digestive tonic, 147-148
Polynesian youth food, 52-53
Polyunsaturated fats as "right" fats, 167
Postgraduate Medicine, 145n
Potato as plant remedy, 64-65
Practice of Respiratory Therapy, 205
Prana for longer youth, 197-206
  for "aging" stomach, 205
  breathing, direction for, 201
    "youth breath" prana, eight steps
        for, 201-203
  and modern science, 203-204

(Prana for longer youth, *cont.*)
reflex functions, rejuvenation of, 206
secret of, 198-199
sitting, proper, Hindu prescription
  for, 200
"total relaxation" program, three-
  step, 200
  benefits of, 200
  as ulcer relief, 204
Pranayama, 198-199 (*see also* Prana for
  longer youth)
Protein, meatless, rice as prime source
  of, 71-72
Protein of soybean and meat, comparison
  of, 161-162

R

Radishes for healing, 65
Raw vegetable juice fast, 36
"Reducing" vitamin, K as, 219-220
Reflex functions, improvement of with
  prana, 206
Reflexology to heal muscular aches and
  pains, 185-196
arms and legs, eight-step way to "forever-young," 193-195
  benefits, 195
benefits of, 187, 190
case histories, 190-193
headaches, relief of, 190-191
hidden scrolls, secrets in, 186-187
motions, eight, 187-189
for wrists and hands, 191-192
Rejuvenation, fasting as traditional
  method of, 32-34
reason for, 37
Religious food, rice as, 71
Resin as ingredient of ginseng, 125
Rice, brown, as most perfectly balanced
  yin-yang food, 29
Rice diet, controlled Oriental, for
  regulation of blood pressure, 70-85
controlled fasting, 85
cooking, Oriental way of, 74-75
fasting programs, ten, 75-85
favored varieties, 73-74
as food of divine health, 71
health benefits of, basic, 71-73
for B-complex vitamins, 72

(Rice diet, controlled Oriental, *cont.*)
calcium, 72
digestibility, 72
low fat, salt, cholesterol, 73
low fiber content, 72
minerals, 72
protein, meatless, 71-72
"Right" fats, 167
Russian Folk Medicine, 118

S

Salt as aid for natural youth, 16 secrets
  for, 129-132
Salt-water soak, for youthful skin, 137-138
Saponin as ingredient of ginseng, 126
Sarsaparilla, 183
Sciatica, relief of, 242
Sea foods, secrets of vitality from, 44-55
  (*see also* Oceans, secrets of Oriental
  vitality from)
Seaweed, how to use, 220
bath, 107-110
  "therapeutic sweating," 108
to control appetite, 221-222
as staple of Orientals, 47
vitamin K concentrated in, 219
Secrets, twelve, for health-building,
  21-24
*Secrets of the Medicine of the Chinese,
  Consisting in Perfect Knowledge of
  the Pulse,* 94
Seed oils, secret power of, 169-170
Self-massage, fingertip, 136
"Self-ventilation" of prana program,
  202-203
Sesame, 181
Sexual power, ginseng as "magic" herb
  for, 114-128 (*see also* Ginseng,
  Korean)
Shakti, 175
Shanghai Sanatorium for Respiratory
  Therapy, 205
Shavasan for increasing oxygen to heart,
  170-173
Shen Nung, Emperor, 56, 176, 226
Shiatsu: secret Japanese finger-pressure
  acupuncture, 93-103
backache, simple programs to relieve,
  98-100

(Shiatsu: Japanese finger-pressure, *cont.*)
  do-it-yourself acupuncture without
    needles, 94-98
  healing power of, secret, 102-103
  how it works, 94-98
  wrists and arms, relief of aching,
    100-102
Shih Ching, 116
Short Version of the Golden Shrine,186
Sinusitis, easing of, 242
Sitting, proper, Hindu prescription for,
  200
Skin, youthful, ocean bathing for, 105
Skin blemishes, prevention of, 237
Skin diseases, herbal healing of, 233
Skin and hair, healthy, secrets of, 129-138
  exercises, 135
  face-lift, herbal, 134
  lemon for natural rejuvenation, 132-134
  salt as natural aid, 16 secrets of using,
    129-132
  self-massage, fingertip, 136
  water treatments, 136-138
    cold-water soak, 137
    salt-water soak, 137-138
Skin rejuvenation, 243
Slimness without dieting, Oriental
  secrets for, 216-225
  appetite, control of with seaweed,
    221-222
  body water, herbs to wash out, 223-224
  diuretic herbs, 223-224
  eating, seven secrets of, 224-225
  honey, 222
  seaweed, how to use, 220
  "slim bath," Hawaiian, 220-221
  steps, nine, 217-218
  vitamin K, 219-220
Smedley, Doree, 210*n*
Soybeans as key to forever-young
  vitality, 153-163
  cooked, increased health benefits of,
    159
  flour, 160
  ingredient, special, 154-156
    for energy, memory improvement,
      steadiness of hands, 156
  "meat without a bone," 154
  and meat protein, 161-162
  milk, 161

(Soybeans, *cont.*)
  nutrients in, 160-161
  "perfect food," reason for
    consideration as, 156-157
  preparation of, 160
  source, meatless, of complete
    protein, 153-154
Starch as ingredient of ginseng, 126
Stomach gas, relief of, 239
Stomach tonic, 237
Stomach upset, apple for, 147
Sunburn, treatment of, 243
Swelling, ointment for reduction of,
  236
*Synopsis of the Technique of Remedial
  Massage*, 190
Szumiao, Dr. Sun, 58, 187, 227

T

Tannin as ingredient of ginseng, 126
Tansy, 183
T'ao Hung-ching, 176, 186
Teas, herbal preferable, 23
Therapeutae, 33
"Therapeutic sweating" in seaweed
  bath, 108
Throat disorders, use of lemon for, 63
Tibetan clove cocktail, 68-69
Tibetan herbs for, healing power of,
  174-184 (*see also* Herbs, Tibetan)
Tissue regeneration through herb Gotu
  Kola, 178-180
Tobacco, fruits as help in easing urge
  for, 151
"Total relaxation" program for prana,
  three-step, 200
  benefits of, 200
Treasury of health secrets and folk
  medicine, 234-243 (*see also* Folk
    medicine)
T'ui-na, 185-196 (*see also* Reflexology)
Tyre, Mysteries of, 33

U

Ulcer distress, prana and, 204
University of Tohoku, 219

V

Vegetable juice fast, 36
Vegetable protein as key to forever-
   young vitality, 153-163
   (*see also* Soybeans)
Versalius, Andreas, 41
Vigor tonic, how to make, 48
Vitamin K, 219-220

W

Water, herbs to wash out of body,
   223-224
Water healers, secret Oriental, 104-113
   for arthritis, ease of, 105-107
   for hair, healthy, 105
   pentagram, mystical, part of, 104
   seaweed bath, use of, 107-110
      "therapeutic sweating," 108
   for skin, youthful, 105
   secret of, 110-112
Water treatments, for youthful skin,
   136-138
Way to Health and Longevity, 217n
Windburn, treatment of, 243
Wormwood, 183
Wrists, aching, limbering up of with
   shiatsu, 100-102

Writings, early Oriental, about Tibetan
   herbs, 176-177
"Wrong" fats, 167
Wu Chung Chich, 177

Y

Yang foods, basic, 24-25
Years Between 75 and 90, 156n
*Yellow Emperor's Classic of Internal
   Medicine*, 20, 116, 186
Yin foods, basic, 24
"Yin-Yang" method, 20-25
   foods, help of to regulate balance
      of, 21-25
   health influences of, 21
   meaning of, 20-21
   yang foods, basic, 24-25
   yin foods, basic, 24
Yoga breathing exercises for increasing
   oxygen to heart, 170-173
   and blood pressure, 171-172
   posture, best, 172
   secrets, two, 172-173
Youth-building power of sea foods,
   51-53
Youth oil elixir, 50